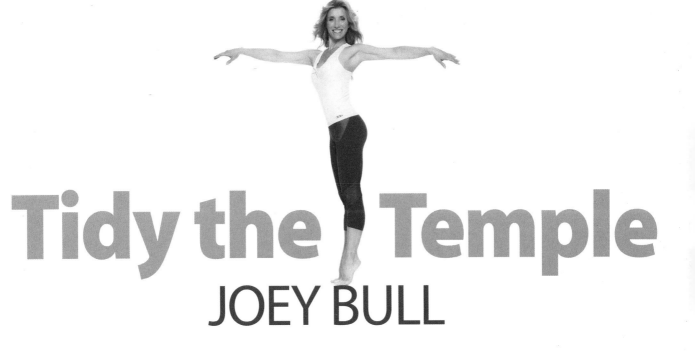

Tidy the Temple

JOEY BULL

Je&E

www.tidythetemple.com

Endorsements

"Joey is a knowledgeable, well informed and talented personal trainer whose expertise of the fitness industry and how to train for best results is unrivalled. She is also a fantastic speaker with a natural talent for inspiring, motivating and encouraging others to get fit – whatever their shape, size or age. Joey makes you believe that getting in the best shape of your life is possible – regardless of your starting point – and she's also one of the most personable and friendly individuals I've met in the business. I can highly recommend her skills and experience."

Christina Macdonald Editor-in-Chief, *Women's Running magazine*

"Joey has experienced and accomplished a vast amount in her life and is a truly inspiring person. Whatever she says or writes on the subjects of health and fitness is always worth hearing and reading."

Rebecca Romero Cycling World & Olympic Champion, *Rowing World Champion & Olympic silver medallist & Ironman World Championship competitor*

"Joey Bull is a leading figure in the UK fitness industry. She has motivated, educated and inspired thousands of people over many years to get fit and lead a healthy lifestyle. I thoroughly recommend *Tidy the Temple* which is a must-read for anyone looking to get fit or looking to improve their fitness."

John Shepherd Publishing Editor of Ultra-FIT Magazine, *GB Athletics Coach & Author*

"Joey Bull is an inspiration to us all and she has opened up her life to us in this book. From her impressive career in the fitness industry she has created *'Tidy the Temple';* a clean and natural regime that will change your life. It is refreshingly honest and down-to-earth. I would recommend this book to everyone, especially those tired of yo-yo dieting and short lived results. Emiko Ray is passionate about food and has been transformed by this regime herself, so who better to write the recipes? She is so practical with her cooking and the recipes are no fuss, easy to follow and simply delicious. These impressive women understand the challenges of every day family life and finding time to exercise and eat healthily and this is why *Tidy the Temple* works so well."

Sarah Leo (née Thomas) *Former international model, now healthy chef*

"As a professional sportsman for over fifteen years I have realised that tailoring my diet towards my health, fitness and training is as important as the actual exercise that I do. *Tidy the Temple* combines both the elements of training and diet, and remarkably the results are visible after just four weeks."

Rob Green *Premiership & England footballer*

Acknowledgements

Guy Holland, who has been instrumental in making this book a reality. For more than a decade he has helped, guided, prompted, cajoled, kick-started and supported. Despite my confusion about what job I have in this world he reminds me and keeps the cogs turning when I haven't been able to.

Rudy de Jong, who has been a rock, a guide, an inspiration and an immeasurable support since my father died. Even in his mid-70s he still knows how to shake a leg and shame the rest of us!

John Dietrich, photographer extraordinaire who has shot me many times over the years and however I've been looking or feeling and whether I've been in a freezing river, up a tree, on dizzying castle ramparts or up a mountain – has always had the skill, patience and humour to make me look my best! Thank you! x

First published in Great Britain in 2013. Text copyright © 2013 Joey Bull

Joey Bull is hereby identified as the author of this work in accordance with the Copyright, Designs and Patents Act 1988.

All rights reserved. No part of this publication may be reproduced, stored in a retrieval system, or transmitted in any form or by any means, electronic, mechanical, photocopying, recording or otherwise without the prior permission of the copyright owner.

Cover design: Peter Hawkes. **Page design and typesetting:** Amanda Carroll / Studio Beam Limited

Cover photos: Andres Lesauvage and Simon Howard. **Photos of Joey:** John Dietrich, Andres Lesauvage and Nigel Harper.

Photos of Emiko: Simon Howard and Joey Bull. **Other photos:** Joey Bull, Emiko Ray, Shutterstock.

ISBN: 9782839907149. Printed and bound in the UK by Butler Tanner & Dennis Ltd, Frome, Somerset.

First Published (2013) by J&E. www.tidythetemple.com

Part 1 *The Tidy the Temple Plan*

Contents

Dedication

To my parents, Peter and Gillian, for making exercise, vegetables and discipline an integral part of my life. To my father for making me touch the finish line on each of our runs or climbs and my mother for being a fine example of vitality in later life. To my dear boy, Oscar, for his endless abundance of joy and irrepressible enthusiasm for life. To his sweet baby brother, Edward, who catapulted me into a new world and wipes my every tear.

4

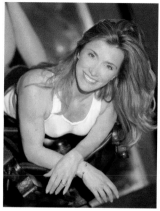

Photo: John Dietrich

A FEW WORDS FROM THE AUTHOR

"Although my background is broad and my experience in health and fitness is extensive, I'm aware there are those who dedicate their lives to researching and re-examining the finest scientific details regarding the body's responses and reactions to all manner of substances, endeavours and environments.

I have had the privilege of meeting and working with some amazing independent research scientists and other very talented people. 'Independent' in the respect that nobody is sponsoring their research or massaging their findings, so I am extremely grateful to have been informed beyond our regular sources.

Like any professional, I have taken the qualifications and covered the theories and research, all of which is worthwhile if only to be able to dismiss some of it as dated or inaccurate. Many valuable discoveries are made in this industry just by being hands-on with a willingness to listen, question, learn and put into practice.

In this book I have combined the best of what I have experienced and used myself for over two decades; with simple facts and positive, efficient results. It is an overall plan of common sense and a healthy respect to self-care.

I have chosen the most effective, honest, achievable and maintainable methods that have crossed my life and packaged it for us, between these covers."

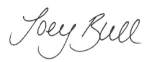

Disclaimer: Not all exercise regimes or eating plans are suitable for everyone. Before starting this programme you may wish to get permission from your doctor to participate in this plan. The advice and instruction in this plan is not intended to be a replacement for medical procedures. Any programme improperly executed can cause injury. The participants of this plan disclaim any liability or loss.

INTRODUCTION

This book contains everything you need to get through the *Tidy the Temple* plan thoroughly: workouts, food lists, recipes, snack ideas, guidance for motivation, goals and preparation tips, daily messages to see you through the 28 days and facts you don't often encounter. Not to mention lots of support – from me and the testimonials of others who've been through this too.

My role is to see you through this step by step, reassure you, keep you on track and make sure you upgrade your body and health in many ways by the end of the first week, not just the last.

It is about supporting the body's system and working with it, rather than challenging its ability to sort out all our bad habits. This will provide a rest for your organs and a tonic for your body. As a result you will be rewarded with the health, shape and condition you've been hoping for.

There are short, effective exercise sessions too that will ensure you'll get the ideal balance between food input and exercise output. These last only minutes and aim to keep every muscle stimulated.

You'll learn quite a lot about yourself along the way too. It is one thing to read theories on which nutrients work for this and that, but another thing to find out for real and feel the benefits. You will be in tune with your body. You'll be fitter and firmer with good energy levels and a neat waistline. Crucially you will also become aware of how you can control cravings.

There will be light information for those of you who just want results and more in-depth information boxes; for those who, like me, always like to know the hows and whys.

We're looking to get the body back in balance where it operates best. To do this we need to get rid of our daily toxins. You may think that your diet has few toxins and your food choices are good but there is always another level that your body could benefit from.

We know that weighing ourselves on the scales isn't a true representation of what shape we're in. You may have come across charts of your 'ideal weight' for your height, age and sex. This is such a general approach and never allows for our differences. We can be fit and heavy, sick and light, fat and light, or heavy and slim. What matters is what we're made up of: a good ratio of muscle density and fat. That is what much of this plan is about.

So we'll purge these toxins, make way for improved cell renewal and make sure that every nutrient we consume gets absorbed. No more hurdling over obstacles in the digestive passage and then fizzling out ineffectively somewhere along the way. It is about clearing the body of foods that inhibit absorption of healthy, cell-recharging nutrients and vitamins, and inhibiting your chances of feeling great and looking gorgeous.

The following chapter has testimonials from several happy clients!

"This is a plan that has worked over and over again for people of all ages, shapes and standards of fitness. It is healthy and effective for fat loss, health, various ailments, water retention and generally looking as vibrant and glowing as you can. Nothing does this better than the combination of good food and exercise."

– Joey Bull

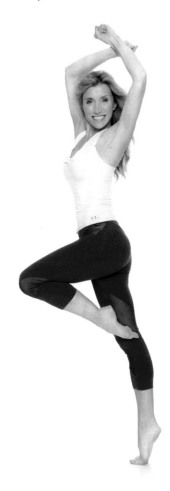

"I couldn't imagine being able to cope for four weeks without caffeine, chocolate, dairy, carbs and my evening glass of wine!"
– Susannah

TESTIMONIALS AND PHOTOS
Susannah's story

"I started Joey's course with mixed emotions. I really wanted to detox my body after a long summer holiday of indulgence but I couldn't imagine being able to cope for four weeks without caffeine, chocolate, dairy, carbs and my evening glass of wine! I have always taken a lot of exercise and the bi-weekly fitness sessions were something I was really looking forward to. Monday morning came and instead of drinking coffee and eating toast it was eggs and herbal tea. Mid-morning snack of tempeh and mung beans felt rather strange and by lunch time I was craving something sweet for pudding, but fruit had to do! I ended up going to bed a lot earlier than normal just so I stopped thinking about the foods I was missing so badly and had the best night's sleep I can ever remember. I guess my body was not having to deal with breaking down any 'toxic' food and was given a break just to rest. I woke in the morning feeling totally refreshed and ready to tackle day 2.

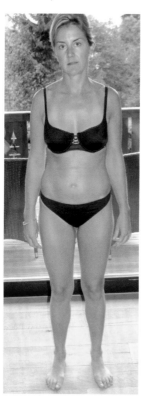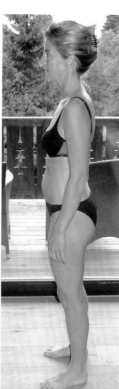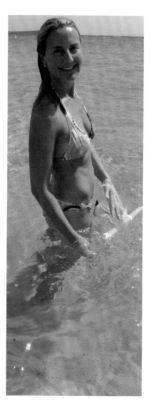

BEFORE

AFTER

The first few days were definitely the hardest and a mild headache on day 3 and slight jitters were a sign of caffeine withdrawal. After that the days slipped by and I managed to get into the swing of my new eating habits. Every night brought me a better and better night's sleep – as deep and undisturbed as I can ever remember – no kicking off the duvet from over heating and no muggy head in the morning.

I lost nearly two kilos in the first week and felt terrific. Everyone commented on my glowing complexion and that only served to fuel my desire to complete the full four weeks and give it my all. The fitness sessions were a mix of weights, cardio and circuit training. Press ups played a large part and I realised that while I thought I was fit I had no upper body strength. This soon changed, however, and Joey managed to slowly build up our strength and stamina.

Joey introduced new foods for us every week which was always a welcome relief as we could expand our culinary efforts and come up with new recipes. Lentils, chickpeas and pulses became brilliant fillers along with butternut and pumpkin. I was never hungry during the four weeks, as is often the case with other diets, and learnt to distinguish between feelings of hunger and craving. As my jeans became looser on me I noticed more important changes – I felt I was on more of an even keel. Before, my emotions and mood seemed to go in swings; on a 'low' I would have a coffee, some chocolate, a glass of wine. Now I was feeling very 'level'; I felt more positive, less irritable and more in control of myself and my moods. It was a wonderful revelation and I loved it!

By the end of *TTT* I felt in the best condition I had for a very long time (physically and mentally). I was happy, healthy, looking good and feeling terrific. A week on, I am finding it hard to return to my old habits and feel that I have been re-educated about what I am putting in to my body and how it will cope. Thank you Joey!"

Susannah

Kathryn's story

"I loved these four weeks, and really appreciate all that you have done for me. You have given me a skill for life, also yes you can print that photo of me grimacing while exercising. At least it shows that I was trying! Best wishes."

Kathryn x

Karina's story

"Dear Joey,

Just finished our last course and it has been so much fun. I did achieve my goals – having thinner legs and a flatter tummy. But I also gained so much more out of it. I know that I can be quite disciplined when it comes to food and I have been able to stand up to the pressure of other people. Even better, I've so much more energy!!! My husband says I'm acting as if on drugs. Must be those hemp seeds!

I've also learned a lot more about nutrition. Especially by eating a little between meals. Because of that I have hardly felt hungry. Also my portion sizes have shrunk. I do think I'll try to keep up with this routine for as much as possible except for when we go out at weekends.

So it has been a great experience. Thanks a lot!!!!"

Karina

"Just finished our last course and it has been so much fun."
– Karina

Pam's story

"Thanks Joey, I hope I'll be in shape after 5 days in Blackpool!!!!!! Harry Ramsden's fish and chips etc, etc … still getting loads of compliments though … thanks to you … saw Sam at the Serenity Salon tonight and she kept asking me how I had lost so much due to your *Tidy the Temple (TTT)*. So glad I can be a good salesperson … you deserve it … as David says … it melts off you with your energetic one minute bursts.

BEFORE

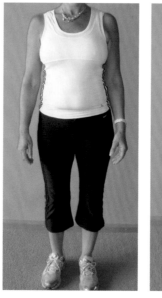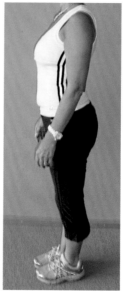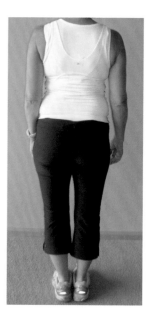

AFTER

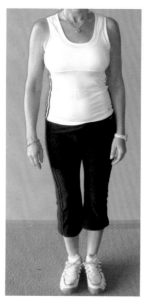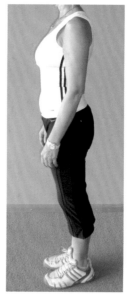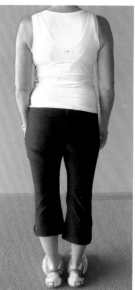

I really meant what I said to you at the sports centre … you are an amazing woman, with an amazing spirit and resilience and you are an inspiration to us all … REALLY."

love Pamxx

Chieko's story

"I had just had a baby and was looking for something that would help me shift the extra baby weight that I was carrying. I wanted a plan that was simple to follow and gave me results. As with anything that challenges a comfy, habitual lifestyle it tends to be the mental rather than the physical side that is harder to overcome; the little negative voice in your head that becomes louder and louder as change starts to take effect. I heard this voice a number of times while I followed Joey Bull's plan but I never gave in to it and I'm so glad I didn't. I believe you receive as much as you put in, and that is true of Joey's *Tidy the Temple* plan.

BEFORE

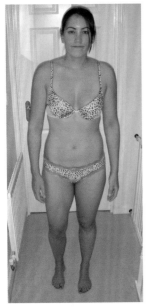
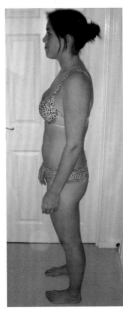
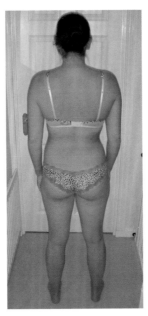

AFTER

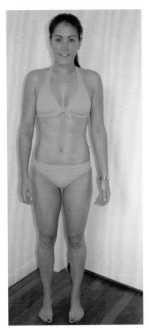
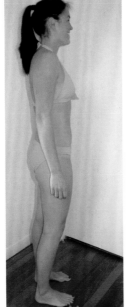
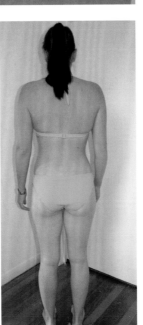

"To cut a long story short, I completed the four weeks and haven't looked back. What a cliche! But it's true."

– Chieko

The first 5 days were the toughest for me, but once I'd overcome the headaches and aches (there were a whole lot of toxins leaving my body!), I started to feel strangely 'clean' inside and had a lot more energy. This vitality was something that I was surprised to receive, but was extremely welcome as I was looking after an 8 month old.

To cut a long story short, I completed the four weeks and haven't looked back. What a cliche! But it's true. I continue to take with me the nutritional themes I have learnt through Joey's plan. The biggest surprise to me is just how effective Joey's plan is. Yes, I lost the baby weight (hooray for me!), but I also gained a healthy, toned body, much more lithe than it had ever been before having a baby – I became a comfortable size 10, whereas pre-pregnancy I was always a size 12. I went on to have another child, and then took on Joey's plan again, to shift the baby weight.

You name a health and fitness plan and I've probably tried it. However, Joey's plan is 'hand-on-heart' the most effective I've ever taken on and continue to follow. Thank you Joey. Joey's *Tidy the Temple* plan is something that I'm so glad I did, and I haven't looked back."

Chieko

Alison's story

"For me, the course has been a real revelation: I can (almost) keep up with the fitness (sometimes!) but have enjoyed trying; I have discovered I like fruit far more than I thought I did and as for juicing – well! I have been hunting high and low on eBay for a reasonably priced juicer as I am amazed how much I even like the vegetable juices!

Thank you for everything you have done for all of us over the past month – I know that you have helped me make a big difference to myself and I know that you have done the same for others too."

Alison Jeffrey

Cecile's story

"With the *Tidy the Temple* plan, Joey forces us to eat lots of fruit and vegetables and the right type of proteins, and forget about all the processed food and industrial rubbish slowly killing us!

The plan lasts for 4 weeks and we do feel better and more energetic for those weeks and lose some weight if needed. But if we keep the good habits, we feel better and much stronger all the time. It is fun to prepare a healthy and colourful breakfast and lunch and dinner and there are certain types of food you don't feel like touching any more because your body itself tells you that it is so bad for it. The plan is educational and so useful!"

Cecile Dargaud

James's story

"I was 10 kg lighter after following the *Tidy the Templ*e recipes. They work wonders for active men too!"

James

BEFORE

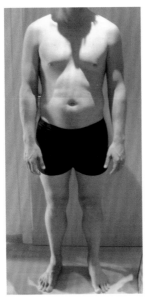 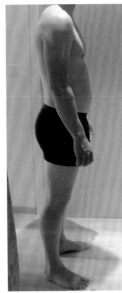 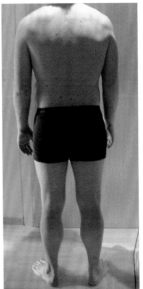

AFTER

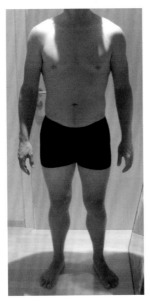 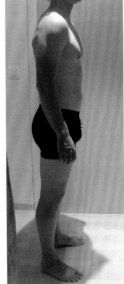 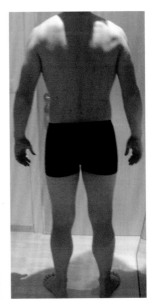

David's story

"Thank you very much for all this – positive stuff and glad it worked! We are finding it hard to go back to our naughty old habits which is a good thing (had a coffee and felt positively wired after it!) so we are doing all we can to squeeze a few more weeks out of our 'healthier' attitude. We so enjoyed *TTT* – thank you for all your hard work, energy and enthusiasm!"

David Anton Smith

"We are finding it hard to go back to our naughty old habits which is a good thing – had a coffee and felt positively wired after it!"
– David

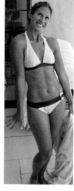

BEFORE   **AFTER**

"The 'Before' and 'After' shots were taken after my babies were born. I have found 'Tidy the Temple' not only helped me get back to my pre-pregnancy shape but my general toning has been better than it ever was before I had children."

– Emiko Ray

Emiko's story

"I love food and enjoy keeping fit but have struggled to find an eating plan that is manageable. This has resulted in times of being very organized and disciplined to longer periods of time doing very little! Joey's *Tidy the Temple* has been a complete revelation to me and I continue to stick to the nutritional advice I have learned over the years from Joey (whilst still sharing her penchant for sweet treats!)

My husband has seen such a transformation in me, not just physically but in my increased energy levels, my decreased mood swings (!) and my general 'glow' that he decided to try *Tidy the Temple* himself. He lost 10 kg by the end of the course and was seeing and feeling the positive effects for himself. "*Tidy the Temple* has changed my life!!!" he concluded. Well I wasn't expecting that! Now our attitude to food has completely changed and we are able, with our children, to experiment with a greater choice of fine foods.

Tidy the Temple is a course that encourages you to eat and not feel hungry. It has opened my eyes to an exciting, positive and refreshing approach to food and has liberated me to exercise for the sheer pleasure and enjoyment of it, as well as knowing that the little exercise space I have is enough to give my body a full workout, using the exercises Joey suggests. It really is a course with minimum input and maximum output.

The 'Before' shots were taken after my babies were born. I have found *Tidy the Temple* not only helped me get back to my pre-pregnancy shape but my general toning has been better than it ever was before I had children. Many of my friends who have taken part have also commented, even over a year on, that they were surprised they have not put the weight back on again. Joey's experience is invaluable and I do not know of a more wholesome, time-saving, common sense and liberating course as *Tidy the Temple* and I wholeheartedly recommend it to you."

Emiko Ray

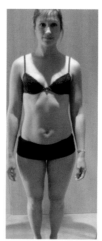
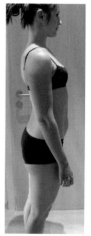
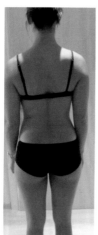
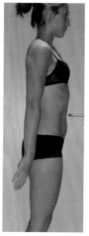
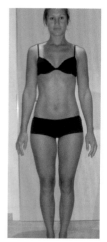
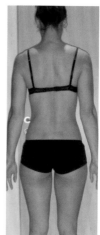

BEFORE   **AFTER**

Helen's story

"Having successfully 'tidied the temple' over these last 28 days it is a great pleasure to write and warmly recommend this course to anyone who fancies a little challenge to their lifestyle with great results. I can honestly say that, since the arrival of my 3 children, I have never found it so easy to get up in the morning!

The recipes were a wonderful aid to the programme – I used them to cook for our family of 5 and just added some potatoes, rice or couscous for the 4 who hadn't voluntarily signed up to the plan! What a great bank of nutritious, straightforward and scrumptious meal ideas – my 2 year old is particularly taken with pomegranate seeds, looking carefully through his salad for the 'sweets'. We were all winners! Thanks so much Joey and Emiko."

Helen Paterson

Alex's story

"I used to be a bit of a gym monkey and have always been sporty yet for the last three years, since becoming a happy father and also having more responsibilities at work, I've had less and less time to keep fit. However, my eating habits didn't change and so I was becoming fat and rather out of shape. I've never been interested in diets as I know that they don't work for me: I'm a high energy person and I need fuel throughout the day. As time went on, and another baby arrived, I had less and less time to myself, less and less time to work out, and I became increasingly unhappy with the way I looked. I was feeling fat, old and heavy. *Tidy the Temple* has been my saviour. I know now that I am in complete control of my weight and also how I look and feel. I lost 11 kgs in 3½ weeks. I love food. I love to cook and the programme has really changed the way I eat throughout the day. My wife and I are now continuing the *TTT* food programme with a day off both mid-week and at the weekend. I now feel much lighter, more energised and most importantly, much younger."

Alex Boyd-Williams

Cobi's story

"Joining and enjoying *Tidy the Temple* works. I did it my own way and it took me two weeks longer. But in the end the whole experience made me stronger and better.

Thank you Joey for your knowledge, understanding and enthusiasm."

Cobi, 69 years

Claire's story

"Thank you for everything. The course has been amazing Joey. You have been such an inspiration to me in so many ways."

Claire Haydock

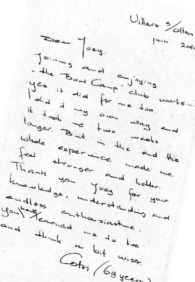

Joey's story

"Since I'd asked others for photos of themselves from before and after the plan, it was only fair that I exposed myself too. These were taken 12 weeks after my second child. I was 43. You can still see the vertical baby line running from top to bottom on my tummy. As you will read later, this was a traumatic and devastating time so I started with my plan soon after the incident so as to help with the emotional stress. Admittedly I wasn't terribly out of shape as I had started eating well after losing Edward to help stabilise hormones and emotions.

BEFORE

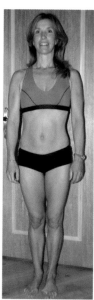 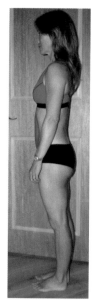 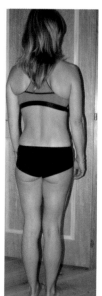 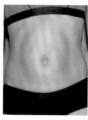

AFTER

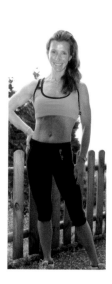 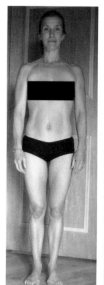 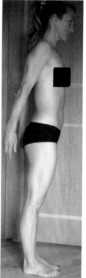 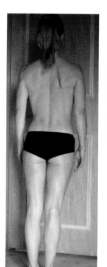 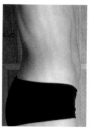

These 'after' pictures show a small difference in size but my body's composition and health was much improved. I needed to be in shape for a DVD shoot so I dropped to a lower weight than ideal so as to allow for the camera's 7 lb gain and wide screen TV!"

– Joey Bull

WHAT TO EXPECT

You can expect to look and feel really well from the inside out.

You can expect an improved body shape and muscle tone, steady moods, (even if you weren't aware you have uneven ones before starting this), your skin will have a healthy glow, feel tighter, look fresher. You can expect healthy insides that shine through on the outside.

If you're prone to small and bothersome ailments, things such as aches, anxiety, poor sleep, feeling run down, you may find these things are diminished, even as early as the end of week one. But there will be another change that might surprise you. Your eating habits and the food that you normally crave or desire, will change. If you pay good attention and keep to the plan, when the 28 days are up, you can expect a **new outlook** on food and your eating habits.

You'll also be more motivated to carry on with exercise.

With the short effective workouts in the exercise section, you'll be able to fit them conveniently into your day and so feel encouraged and motivated to keep the ball rolling.

Over a short duration, there can be so much healing, correction and rebalancing going on.

Some days you'll feel it and notice it, other days it'll just be happening behind the scenes. It is believed that for every year of sickness it takes one month of correction. One month? After all that time of accumulated 'mistakes', errors and the odd bad habit, that is fast work.

You may not be sick but all of us can improve our health rapidly and realistically, thoroughly and healthily, during a single month.

During these days you'll learn a lot. Not just about eating and exercising but about how well your body and mind can respond to good self-care.

In addition you'll learn the difference between:

- hunger and cravings
- weight loss and fat loss
- a healthy body and one that is simply getting away with it!

MY STORY

My family were keen 'exercisers'. Not the indoor type but the walking-through-wet-hills type.

We spent most of our holidays in soggy tweed breeches marching up mountains for windy picnics on summits somewhere. I think we conquered all the British ones but I was the least enthusiastic among the five of us and so have no recall of the peaks' names. I rebelled from this hardy life and took up ballet. It was the being indoors, in insulated studios that appealed to me. I would escape into the fantasy of dance and music, ignorant of the fact that I'd actually stepped from one hardy hobby into another.

Nonetheless, I was immersed in full-time dancing school, flanked with holidays back in the wet mountains. Dancing was my life and income until one day in my mid-twenties I had a ski accident. I ruptured three ligaments in my knee, and my lower leg dragged behind me uselessly. Pirouetting and pretty jumps were over in a flash and I spent my time in hospital post-op wondering what on earth I was going to do.

Having not dedicated my education days to useful subjects like science and maths, but to just ballet, the thought of starting over was overwhelming and extremely disappointing. So, I didn't. I just ignored what the prognosis was, ignored the 'you'll never be able to' list and buckled down to some serious rehab. It was for me, the easiest way out, 'just try harder' seemed to be the only thing I really knew.

Within a year I was fit, not perfect pirouette fit but I could bluff the rest. And bluff I did. I entered my first UK fitness competition and was placed 4th. It wasn't my scene but, after mountains and ballet, this was manageable. The next year I won the UK Miss Fitness title and went out to the international circuit. I was up against the big girls there and they were big, thanks to their 'performance enhancement' help, or steroids as you and I know them. Unless I played their game I'd never make the top three so after placing 8th in the World, I left the international scene and came home to compete. I scooped up 3 more UK titles.

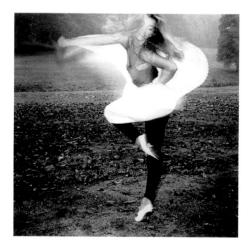
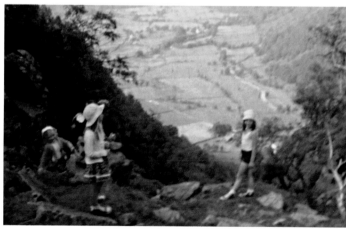

Somehow word got out that I was more than a fitness chick and I could paddle canoes and climb rocks. I was invited to join the British team for a World Expedition adventure race in Borneo. I'd been to Borneo and I knew what this meant. 500 kilometres of slopping through jungles, rivers and leeches, with heavy rucksacks. It was worse than that though, there was no time for sleep except slumped over your canoe paddle, between strokes. We spent 10 days awake, running on adrenaline, eating lard and jelly beans. The parasites loved us and we returned home infested with them. The next invitation was to race in Fiji. I skipped the offer.

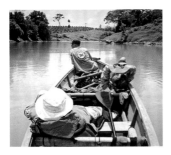

Shaping up for fitness competitions used to be a large part of my discipline. The competitions were divided into three parts: one of a pure fitness test, the next more of a creative gymnastic style performance; and the last, and my least favourite, judging our body shapes. Were they athletic, feminine and balanced?

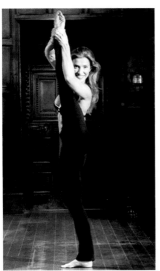

Photo: Nigel Harper

I was a keen eater and loved my cakes but, in 'shaping up season', my midnight feasts stopped. We'd train hard, cut out fun food and live a life of broccoli, fish and rice. Then in the last few days before competing, not even rice. It wasn't healthy and I know better now, but in shape we were. Our bodies were tight but our faces tired, and keeping in top shape like that, was unsustainable after a few days. But of course we timed things perfectly for competition date and forensic scrutiny! The demand and expectations were unusually high and so maintaining this level year long wasn't realistic.

Out of competition, or 'off season' as they'd say, we were fit but didn't look particularly good from it. It seemed like we were a bit stodgy or bulky 'off season'. Yet in prime competing time we'd be in great shape with tiny waists but rather drawn in the face. That was always the downside. Tweaking the diet was key to getting the look just right. That is, eliminating some foods or gorging on others. It even went as detailed as 'if it's red, don't eat it', not even a tomato! The timing of knowing what to eat and when to eat it, was impeccable. We knew how to shape up, slim down and fill out in perfect time for championship day. And, if you had your eyes on the trophy, you'd pull out all the stops, and eat to win.

The learning curve

Over 23 years on and it's clear that the way we used to 'eat to win' is unsustainable! Like many people, I love my food and I could race any of you to the dessert trolley a few times over. But gorging like a Roman full-time isn't fun and our mood and motivation flattens. When it isn't even a treat any more it is time to take stock. When I am drawn to processed foods, white bread and a fluffy Victoria sponge and think nothing of it, I know I need sorting out. Looking in the mirror and catching a fold of flab here and there, a spongy textured skin, flat complexion and a less than perfect temperament looking back at me, I know it's time to get on top of it.

I can't spend all year being wonderfully healthy and being resistant to goodies or baddies, but I can for a few months in that year. So can you, it's just that we need a kick start, a change of state, a boot up the backside and then habits will change for the better for quite a while, and we will be better for it. Days, weeks and months of improved habits, over time, add up to years. What a difference that makes to your wellbeing, removing disease and rotten ailments. Any worries you had about being sore or poorly can be ditched, because ailments can't grow or breed so well in a bonny body.

The occasional bad habit won't kill you, but an accumulation of a frequent few will certainly do you no good.

My personal point and life's big challenges

I am writing this section of this book just twelve weeks from having given birth to my second baby. I held baby Edward the full term of nine months. Tragically, due to a 'true knot' in his umbilical cord just centimetres from his belly button, he died during labour. The knot tightened as the waters broke and he suffocated. It was a rare tragedy of 1 in 2,000 babies. Statistics mean nothing when they hit you though. I had a perfectly healthy baby that died on what should have been one of the best days of my life.

Most women consider childbirth to be the biggest event of their life and possibly the most painful thing. But this was an experience that was beyond natural childbirth. Back-to-back contractions ripped my womb more and more until it burst. Soon there was no longer a wall of protection between Edward, the placenta and I, we were all one soup together. Despite my pleas for surgery, the ripping went unrecognised while the nurses and medics dithered with other duties. Clearly I was no longer a priority and was left for an over-long labour in this mess. I lay in silence coping with the pain, there was no energy to scream, talk or shed tears. I had to shut down while the rest of me broke down.

A day later an emergency C-section was agreed and the trauma was uncovered; my previous C-section from 4 years before had split open, taking with it further tears up the womb, its contents burst into my abdomen. Thank goodness our dear baby wasn't alive to suffer it. While other mums were fussing and loving their newborns, I was still searching for mine. Losing a child is a parent's biggest fear and here I was living it. Hormones, instinct and nature were working against me, my body didn't know my baby had died and it carried on as if I still had one. My world was turned upside down. The only thing that wasn't in tatters was his little room that we had prepared and furnished with a new cot and cupboard full of baby clothes.

A full-term pregnancy, a healthy baby, the expectation, the hope, a new baby room, other home adjustments, an excited family … a ruptured womb, a Caesarean and worse, all of this for nothing. This was followed by months of recovery and nights of sleeplessness, with no baby for company, no Edward to make it worthwhile as he was not there to blur the trauma or to colour in my life. Having a baby is the biggest emotional high, losing a child is the other extreme.

Often the desire of a new mum is to get more sleep and to get her figure back. My desires weren't as detailed or futile. I just wanted my baby back. I still do.

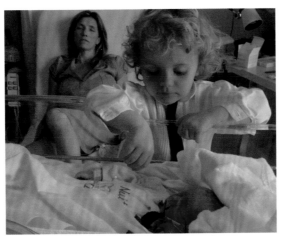

Oscar admiring his brother. He saw through the bruises and blood and became instantly attached to him

Motivation to work or to work out was non-existent, everything seemed fatuous and without substantial meaning, apart from of course my other treasured child, Oscar. Everything I had learned, practised and believed in was surrounded by doubt, especially health, fitness and faith. It was a time of profound reflection.

It threw a lot of questions up in the air too. I had a healthy baby, I was healthy, I paid attention during pregnancy to mother's and baby's best needs, but my baby still died. What, I asked, did health and fitness really serve, when fate at its cruellest takes over?

So *can* health and fitness serve something even after such desolation? It couldn't change my outcome but it can change my perspective, my mood and therefore my perception, it can expose me to a prettier view, rather than being under my blanket of gloom. And from this prettier perspective I can find happier roads between broken bridges. Maybe too, if I am lucky, I will have a third baby. It won't be sweet Edward but it will be a blessing. (See 'The Turnaround', page 156).

It was a lot to go through and if there was ever a time I needed to be gentle with myself it was now. All those jabs and drugs they gave me in hospital, all those things I hate, the sadness, the tension, the physical butchering … none of it is the making for a happy healthy body. And a healthy body is what I needed to help see myself through the first stages of this agony.

Physically, I was so restricted from my operation, and not being able to move is always depressing. But I sat it out, feeling the pain and crying myself dry. I didn't force anything – discipline, diet, exercise, anything. I let it all be. Then as the inertness began to fade I realised my body deserved healing attention, and a tour of the tea shops wasn't achieving that. This body needed all the help I could provide it with: 'tidying the temple' was in order.

And that is what works best for all of us. So I got back on track and cleaned up, shaped up and perked up and, if after all of this I can pull my finger out, I hope you can too!

You've got the book, now make sure it is money well spent.

WHY TIDY THE TEMPLE?

There are plenty of eating plans, diets, promises that we encounter in shops, online, in magazines, on TV and in clubs. It is the same the world over.

Some might leave you feeling hungry, create wind or give you smelly breath. Some might get the weight off courtesy of water loss and muscle depletion, then just add it back on again with interest. So how do you know which one will serve you best?

Having been in the fitness industry for more than 23 years (which is quite a while bearing in mind how young the modern health and fitness industry is!), I've seen a lot of products, plans and gimmicks come and go. Admittedly some things fail from poor marketing resources and others, contrarily, do extremely well. What has been very evident over this time is that it isn't necessarily the good quality or truly effective things that make the shelves and headlines, but the hyped up, sensationalised and well-marketed.

Beware of false claims

Something that has troubled me is the extravagant and spurious claims made in the health and fitness industry, often accompanied by a big price tag. More commonly than not, I've seen the beginnings of these products and plans, the scientific research behind them and then the sales tools and launch that follows. The stories and claims can be greatly extended and rather incongruent to the original material and truth. But we can't blame them. Business is business. It is up to the consumer to be discerning and informed.

If only we could 'lose ten pounds in ten days' or shape up 'effortlessly', but we can't. Sure we can lose lots of weight but what is that weight made up of? Water? Muscle? Some fat? Any wonder then when someone has been to diet club, they keep going to diet club? So many, especially ladies, seem to be permanently on a diet, counting calories or points and then, when they come off their diet, the weight piles back on. And so it continues. That is no way to live, surely? How much more evidence do you need to realise that what you are doing is not truly effective? You'd hardly keep taking your car to the same garage if it ended up running worse when you collected it!

Keeping it sensible and achievable

We are bombarded with mixed messages, different fads, different styles or tricks trying to achieve the same thing. But the answer is so simple, keep the body in healthy balance and it will do the rest. It isn't about restriction of intake but the quality and regularity of food.

So this is what makes *Tidy the Temple* common sense. There are no tricks, bluffs and no attempt to con the very intelligent functions of the body. The body is very smart. The best we can do is support it, work with it and give it what we can, to get more out of it. Give it a break from challenge and give it a chance over these 28 days to show you how good things can get.

Keeping it healthy in the long-term

Having worked with many people with an interest in improving their health and fitness, I'm at the sharp end of what works and what doesn't. I've also spent years applying theories to myself before putting them on others and seeing the variation on how mine and their bodies respond.

During my international competitive years in fitness, it was clear to see what worked long-term and what worked for the short-term. I saw what got competitors through an event and the contrast between when they were 'off season' or between competitions or races. We could manipulate how our bodies looked within a few days with some drastic dietary tweaks. But these weren't lasting results, not to mention healthy or even manageable long-term.

More information Weight gain after dieting

So why does that happen? Is it the individual's lack of willpower? Sometimes yes, but given the right food choices in the first place, willpower wouldn't be an issue. What other reason could it be?

Restrictive diets confuse the body

Think of it like this. A restrictive intake of food actually confuses a hormone in the brain called the fat set point. If the body has a marked reduction in food intake, the body's energy output slows down to accommodate the reduction. If someone is used to consuming 3,000 calories per day of a mix of all sorts, to suddenly reduce that consumption by half or even a third, will cause havoc with the fat set point. And this will be in the form of slowing down metabolism to handle the shock. If it is used to 3,000 calories, to give it 2,000 for a duration of time will cause the body to hang on to fat for reserves, just like a creature going into hibernation.

Weight from fat is harder to shift

In such a diet or calorie reduction, the body may shed weight, a lot of weight, but fat will be its last choice. That is one reason why when the diet is over, the weight piles back on. Why? Because the kilos of weight lost, weren't all fat. Fat takes time to mobilise and leave, just as it takes time to be laid down or return. On the other hand muscle and water weight is fast to leave and water is fast to return.

Resetting the fat point

Another reason why, after some diets, the weight piles back on is a very key one. After a reduced calorie diet, the fat set point has been reset, only to a lower level … than ever before. That means you can't eat as much as before, even before this whole weight problem thing started. Now the body is clocking anything coming in over the set point as excess fuel. So to lose more fat, you'd have to reduce your intake even more to get success.

So by now, you are barely eating anything and still have a weight problem. We've all seen some big people eat much less than other smaller ones yet continue to struggle with their weight. Doesn't seem fair does it? But until the fat set point hormone is back to its efficient rate, this continues.

Only, no one tells the dieter this! Instead the dieter will blame him or herself, not the plan or guidance they've been given. There are many out there who feel quite disillusioned about their weight or condition. There can also be a sense of failure for this recurring issue and lack of long-term success.

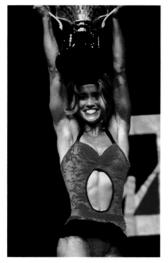

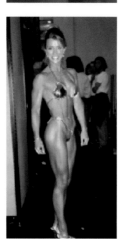

PERSONAL POINT

For my part I gave it my all with diet and fitness and I realised my natural limits.

So I retired from competing at 8th place worldwide with 4 British titles, rather befuddled. To raise my game would have meant getting involved in choices that went against my whole ethos. My belief was health and fitness, and ideally on the back of that I'd win the trophy.

Others' sole focus was the trophy, no matter what it meant to their bodies. I believed many actually compromised their health for that trophy. I didn't know at the time how few of us were 'clean', meaning using no sports enhancing drugs, human growth hormone or fat burning substances. I was shocked when I found out later. I should have spotted the less than 'clean' symptoms of my fellow competitors but I was innocent to the 'look' that left its trace on some athletes. They were things we'd joke about: wide jaws, big noses, spotty skin … looking back there was plenty of that. And although my nose is no button, it is from my father's side and not from a cocktail of sports improvers!

It wasn't until we all went out to eat after my last international championship that the penny dropped. The world reigning champion at the time, lovely as she was, shook her handbag and some pills fell out. It was my savvy mate who recognised them as amphetamines: 'Nothing serious though, just standard stuff,' she said.

Naturally, I felt 'had', fooled and stupid. I'd gone the really long way round to get in shape. I didn't even trust protein shakes for fear of what might be masked within and suppressed by the marketing hype.

Though I have to admit to the satisfaction of finding out after I'd left the competitive circuit that I'd beaten some who'd 'cheated'! Years on I've seen those same figures and faces, quite changed, a little weathered … and not for the better. I can't see if their health is affected or how these things manifest long-term but all we do know is that you can't buy health and fitness, you just have to do it yourself.

The starting point is always difficult. How much exercise should I do, how little should I eat, what is best to eat and what can I get away with? It isn't always straightforward and we can get lured by great packaging and advertising claims. What does not help are all the labels of low fat this and that, the slimmer's choice or 'healthy' slapped across products. What does help is to read the labels and know for yourself.

There are plenty of options out there for diets, plans, healing and more, and many of them no doubt, are very good. But this plan will keep you informed, motivated and take care of you until you can take care of yourself, effortlessly, inside and out.

The food choices, eating habits and exercise all combine to offer a full shaping up, healthy package. It is a respected method among trainers and nutritionists. There are no tricks, replacement meals, supplements or manufactured merchandise. It is designed to work with the body and support it. It is just pure good eating with exercise sessions designed to work all the muscles, improve the heart's capacity and, very importantly, in a conveniently short space of time.

So it won't be time consuming. Not many of us have time for an hour's exercise a few times a week, especially if work and family commitments play a part in controlling your lifestyle. This is to help you find more time, more energy and get the health and fitness things sorted. Just make sure you get organised in the first few days and it'll help enormously with getting into the swing of the new habits and, therefore, optimise all your efforts.

You'll be clearing out, cleaning up, toning up and brightening up. Getting health from the inside out.

It goes back to basic food that assimilates well with us. Plus exercises that not just boost great muscle condition, but your body's metabolism, the machine that burns our fat and fuel.

As I say to my groups; "After all we're not just looking to shape-up! We want vitality and better concentration. We want our bodies charged with health and energy, with tight and plump skin, luscious locks and nice nails! Not to mention bright eyes and bushy tails!"

There is a small downside. You may feel a bit tired, even get a bit shaky or feel unwell for a few days. But dig deep and keep going … that is when you can be sure of becoming healthier, leaner and sparkle with more energy and vitality than ever before. Remember, for every year of bad habits or with sickness, it takes one month for correction.

Let's get started …

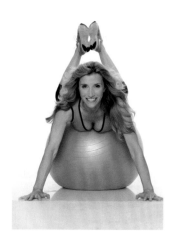

EXERCISE

As previously stressed, nothing gets great results better than the combination of well chosen exercise and well chosen food. There are a variety of exercise options out there these days and they all serve something. The most important thing is to get moving and make it a regular habit. But for time restrictions and getting a whole body workout, this needs more thought.

Four exercise routines have been worked out for the *Tidy the Temple* plan and are illustrated from page 91. They take between 12 and 15 minutes. Obviously, the more you get the hang of them, the more time efficient they will become. They allow for warming up time, working each muscle and working the heart gradually and efficiently over the minutes.

Generally each exercise should take 30 to 40 seconds. They are a mix of resistance exercises, meaning using your muscles more, and movements that will get your heart and lungs pumping. It may not be what you're used to but give it your best. Start with the level you feel appropriate for you (see the chart on page 25) and don't be afraid to step it up a level. These sessions are short and won't leave you feeling shattered or over-exercised. Instead you'll feel recharged, like you've worked all over but still have plenty more energy for your other errands ahead of you.

More information Short, sharp workouts

It used to be thought that for exercise to be worthwhile we should plod away running or on a stepper, or other apparatus for 30 minutes. And many of us did, often for longer. The only thing was, that past the initial adjustment time of getting into exercise, there didn't seem to be any visual changes. Yet we were too scared to stop in case we 'lost our fitness' or form. The other problem was, after weeks or months, most people gave up while their gym membership carried on.

Fortunately for most of us, there is a lot of evidence to support that workouts can be short and sharp and bring great results for improving form and fitness. This is something I've advocated for years. Not just because it is time effective but also because of better results. It is much less draining on the immune system, works better for avoiding wear and tear on joints and sparks up the metabolism, therefore burning energy very effectively all day long. It isn't the time exercising

that counts, but the accuracy of the choice of exercises and effect that has on the heart's range. All of this makes a difference to the body's recovery, fitness and how long you'll burn fuel post workout.

Optimising the given time you have for exercise is vital if you don't want to waste time and effort. In this case the exercises are selected for maximum muscle stimulation and cardio output during a few minutes. Therefore it is important that the heart rate increases steadily from your starting exercise and then is taken up and down throughout the workout. These workouts take care of that. If you were to see your heart's activity on a graph it would look like pointy summits of a mountain range with peaks and dips. It is this that greatly improves the heart muscle yet, with the lows in between, allows for recovery, and for you to gather the energy for the next peak of exertion.

This way of exercising makes sure that you get the best out of a short but complete workout.

THE WORKOUTS

The Starter's Workout

Pick this workout if:

- your activity levels are low other than home chores
- you are active, a regular walker or jog occasionally
- you used to exercise but haven't in a while

Intermediate

Pick this workout if:

- you go to exercise classes or follow your own home workout
- you are used to physical activity, albeit your work
- you feel comfortable with short runs

Experienced Exerciser

Pick this workout if:

- you are a regular exerciser and used to resistance work

If you are injured or recovering from time out for one reason or another, the starter's workout will be suitable for this. The moves are energetic but not strenuous and are very low impact to joints.

The Filler Workout

Pick this workout to:

- add between other workout days as your fitness improves

What will I need?

There is an exercise session designed for no equipment at all, so either way, with or without kit, you can have a good workout.

BUT … if you have some small hand weights, they would be ideal. Even an exercise band works for these exercises. But don't let a lack of equipment delay your start date! Just dig out heavy things from around the house or your larder:

- heavy tins
- flour bags
- logs from the fire's stash
- heavy books that you can get your grip around
- bottles of wine, or fill up bottles with water, add sand if you have some!

Try to use 1.5 litre plastic bottles for the extra weight. Remember that 1 litre of fluid weighs one kilo.

Space wise you'll barely need any. So long as when you throw your hands upwards you don't touch the ceiling, as little as 1 metre by 2 metres of clear floor space will suffice. If there's more space, use it, but the important thing is to get the workouts done. Save moving chairs and furniture around for cleaning days!

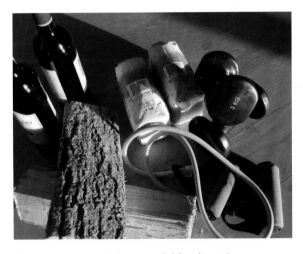

How much weight would be best?

Assuming you are injury free:

- For ladies: 1 kilo minimum for each hand, ideally 2.5 kilos each hand, 3 to 4 kilos if you are used to weight training.
- For men: minimum 3 kilos but ideally 4 to 5 kilos each hand.

When is best to work out?

This depends on your daily routine of course but, for fat loss purposes, it is most beneficial to exercise after fasting, i.e. before breakfast. However this is not the time to get your fastest athletic times or personal best performances!

How does the body burn more fat?

Put simply like this … the meals you eat get digested and then stored as glycogen in the muscles. Glycogen provides us with instant energy. The glycogen levels are richer if they are made up of the type of food mentioned in the 'What won't I be eating' paragraph on page 37. So if we reduce those foods, we reduce the levels and therefore put more demand on the body to find energy from elsewhere, in this case the fat cells.

However, if you were to greatly reduce your calories and intake of food, the sequence would be different. The body would draw energy from the least important tissue required for survival, ie muscle. In doing this, the body is effectively eating itself and we call this a cannibolic state.

It is very important to eat sufficiently and frequently to avoid this. Going hungry is getting it wrong. For everyday purposes, muscle is a valuable tissue. It is fibrous, has blood flow, increases circulation and is a demanding tissue. Its existence, without even being exercised, means the body burns more calories, more fuel and more fat.

So imagine how much more it can burn with exercise. Much of this plan is about keeping muscle and putting demand on it, so as to create improved muscle density and tone. The short workouts in the exercise section are designed for this.

So, we are feeding muscle and reducing the fat storage.

Can I burn fat just around my backside or midsection?

No, it doesn't work like that. The fat the body draws on is from the cells all over the body. It then goes via the liver before being used as energy. However, from observation of many cases, visually fat tends to go from where it was most recently laid down.

With this plan, we are looking to mobilise fat from storage in the fat cells rather than use the simple sugar energy (glycogen) stored in the muscle cells. Drawing on energy from the fat cell is a slower process than our usual surge of energy stored in muscles, this is why feeling a little lacking in energy isn't unusual within the first few days of *Tidy the Temple*.

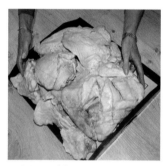

Volume of fat

The fat pictured here weighs 2 kilos (4.4 pounds). Unlike muscle, fat isn't dense and takes up a lot of space spreading out over the body. This shows you the significant size of only 2 kilos of fat.

If this was 2 kilos of muscle, it would be one third of this size.

Much more information Exercise levels

It isn't your age or sex that should determine your efforts, but your history of exercise and present activity levels.

Your heart rate is also a huge indicator of the intensity that is best to follow. Despite common belief, this can't be generalised by age or sex either. There are plenty of 20-year-olds who would find maintaining 150 heart beats p/m extremely tough, and there are plenty of 70-year-olds who'd find 150 BPM easy.

This is something I've observed over the years. Everyone is different and there can be no general rule for an age group, male or female. To generalise like that can leave people either de-conditioned, over trained or worse, rather unwell. But unfortunately it is easy to be misled, as this is the information that is plastered all over fitness equipment and leaflets, no matter the quality of the product.

It could be that you have two people of the same age, sex and who even share the same sport. One could have a maximum heart rate of 150 BPM, the other of 220 BPM. Put in the same race the only one with the advantage will be the one who is fitter. That needn't necessarily be the one who has trained the most, but the one who has trained most effectively.

Rather like the size of our feet and many other things, heart rates are genetic. And whatever we have,

serves us fine. It doesn't mean that fewer or more beats per minute is better or worse, improves performance or lessens it. It means, just as it would with a pair of shoes, that is our size. The best we can do is work accordingly with it and optimise its potential.

If we wanted to get exact and really understand what works best in getting the ultimate workout heart rate wise, then physical tests give the answers. With this information it is possible to know how best to train, for how long, in which range of heartbeats and, get really fit without draining the body. Many people think more is better with workouts but this method proves otherwise.

Working with this information in mind will give you much more confidence about your exercise sessions. You'll soon become in tune with your fitness ability and limitations and know how to exercise extremely effectively to suit these. Best of all, over time, you will understand more about your heart's beats and its indications, than any trainer or doctor could tell you.

To get the best out of the workouts in the exercise section, aim for around level 6 to 7 of exertion for the more intensive exercises. There will be a natural recovery during the less demanding exercises.

Assessing your level of exertion

Since the information and testing isn't widely available, the next best thing is to go by how you feel during your workouts. On a scale of 1–10 you could estimate your exertion. It could be something like this:

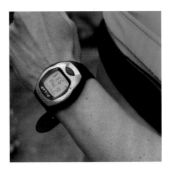

- ■ 1 Easy walking, as if walking around town
- ■ 3 Comfortable for the heart and lungs, maybe starting to perspire lightly
- ■ 7 Quite a lot of effort, not so comfortable and would like to slow down soon
- ■ 10 Fast panting, can't get enough oxygen, not feeling good, may blackout

Naturally the output for what it takes to feel any of these levels will change over time with progress. Walking your local hill may feel like around number 7 now but after a couple of weeks or more, it could be a comfortable 3.

HOW WILL I FEEL?

Side effects

There may be some side effects during the first few days of this cleanse. Just let them be and sit them out. They will be indicators that your body is getting rid of rubbish because now, finally, it can spend time doing that, rather than busying itself filtering the rubbish we usually consume. Symptoms may include headaches, spots, rashes, a change of bowel movement, the shakes and possibly aching joints.

Whatever they are, be sure that it isn't because you're poisoning yourself with healthy food. Be confident these are things coming to the surface and leaving. Let it all be, let it all pass naturally and don't even consider reaching for the painkillers. What would your liver think of that as an option?

Why these side effects?

See it like a war. The enemy invades, infrastructure falls apart and everything goes into emergency mode. That's us when we're carrying on with bad and somewhat toxic habits. Then when it is all over, the enemy leaves but there is still a trail of devastation that comes out in all sorts of ways. That's us as we clean up and detox.

Only we fix faster than post-war problems. What really happens is that while we're carrying on with our less than healthy habits, the white blood cells (the soldiers) go into emergency mode and deal with the immediate problem, e.g. sorting out poor food choices, substances and the resulting reactions. If we keep to a healthy diet and there are no challenges in the foods we digest, the white blood cells won't be on overload and can get on with their regular doings, like dealing with the body's natural day-to-day self-correction. This is when there may be more obvious signs of purging toxins, like through the skin, short-term aches or just feeling different.

More of these examples will be mentioned in the daily messages.

Further side effects

You may also realise how reliant you have been on highs from stimulants such as coffee, alcohol, sugar and other starchy food, even if you feel your intake of these things is moderate. Your new habits could even make you realise what an addict you've been!

It is very important to trust in the first few days that you don't 'need' that coffee and the body will balance itself out, for the better, without it! Soon you will be self-reliant and later on, any 'hit' will feel like over-kill. The plan may even throw up any beliefs you had on being healthy before, especially if you have put your faith in diet products or manufacturers' claims over the years.

Remember this is a clean up. It is short-term and sticking to it for the duration will get you back on an even keel. The emphasis is on these 28 days. There is a section on 'Moving On' from this 28 day plan on page 145.

The upsides

One of the best parts of this plan is how, afterwards, people see things differently. It becomes clear how our eating habits affect our moods and thoughts, motivation and energy. Already significant differences before you even jump on the scales or try on your old jeans. Reading the testimonials makes it clear how much of an unknown bonus this was for previous participants.

It sounds like a big claim but it makes sense. What we fuel ourselves with makes a difference to how we feel. How we feel makes a difference to how we view things. It took me a long while to realise (and longer to admit it), that a binge of cakes and sugar not only leaves me feeling lethargic but rather timid, sensitive and paranoid.

Another huge mental side to this is knowing you can pull it off. By that, I mean you and your well-balanced body and mind are in control. You will no longer be making decisions or choices coming from fancies, cravings or just the same old habit. Having mental clarity means having a better grasp on things.

Seeing the potential that your body has, given half the chance to correct itself, is extremely rewarding. The only thing is us humans don't always appreciate what we have until it is gone. So make sure you take 'before' and 'after' photos so you can see objectively for yourself. Try the little tests too from the section on page 30. These are little ideas that will confirm your progress beyond clothes feeling looser and vitality feeling stronger!

Then of course there is the obvious: you'll look and feel great, you'll look and feel healthier, your body will have had a taste of how great it could be without years of titbits or even abuse! Now take off a layer and think of the changes that will be occurring within. The cells would have had much improved conditions for regeneration and everything and anything related to circulation and nutrients will be rested and rejuvenated.

The treats you used to relish will hold a different meaning. Years of using them as a comfort, a crutch or quick pleasure will change now. Wouldn't you rather leave these debilitating habits behind? We hang on to them like a comfort blanket yet they serve nothing at all. A few seconds of delight for a formation of a habit that does nothing other than de-condition us and get us on a roll of being unhealthy. Why not just shine and feel your best, all the time?

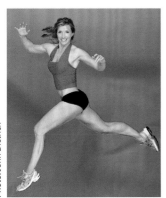

Photo: John Dietrich

Your body will have had a taste of how great it could be without years of titbits or even abuse!

BEFORE YOU GET GOING
Try These Tests

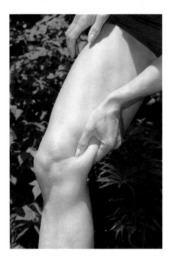

Tummy shake

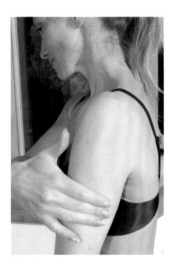

Knee pinch

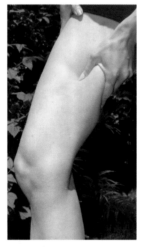

Upper leg

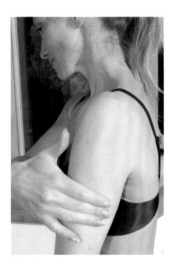

Arm brush

1. Tummy shake

Stand in front of a long mirror, pull up your clothes to expose your tummy and start jigging or jumping. Keep an eye on that tummy and then stop moving suddenly, does it shake about?

Yes? This shows that you are carrying excess water. This doesn't mean you are over hydrated but that the cells are carrying water. The cells draw in water to buffer a chemical imbalance.

2. Knee pinch

Roll up your trousers and on the inside of the knee, between fingers and thumb, grab the flesh to the side of the joint. Give it a bit of a squeeze, does that feel a little sore or sensitive?

Yes? This is normally an indication that the lymphatic (your drainage system) is on overload.

3. Upper leg

On your inner thigh, about half way down towards your knee, grab a handful of flesh and squeeze it tight. Does it look rather dimpled and uneven? Yes? Cellulite as we know it has been the bane of women's lives for decades. For all the potions that may be out there, nothing has ever been as successful for ridding cellulite from my ladies and I, as keeping to this plan.

4. Arm brush

On the upper part of the back of your arms, feel if this is smooth or not. Try the upper, outer side of the legs too. Is it a little rough and bumpy? This can be an indication of poor absorption of nutrients or a lacking of certain nutrients.

5. Face

Look at your face, your complexion, note its colour and luminosity, do you have bags under your eyes?

6. Tongue

Now look at your tongue, note the colour, does it have a white coating, are there any cracks or prominent lines?

7. Heels

Take a look at your heels, are they smooth or very dry with deep cracks?

8. Liver stroke

On the right side of your tummy, with two fingers, brush across outwards with light pressure from the centre of your tummy, just below your ribs, to about belly button level. We're trying to follow the liver. Watch the marks your fingers leave. Do they leave a trail at all? Is there a whitish mark that stays a second or two? This trail can indicate whether the liver is on overload or not.

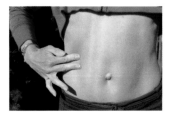

Liver stroke

Get started 'tidying your temple'

Fix a date with yourself as to when you're going to start 'tidying your temple'. Come up with all the reasons you want to feel great, override excuses and other hurdles. What can really stop you from pulling this off? You! So dig deep, have a talk with yourself and tighten those reins. You are going to sort this from the inside-out. What are a few weeks in your life to committing to a healthier more energised and vibrant life? Nothing! As we used to say in expedition races when we were wounded and weathered. "Dry your eyes and crack on". Get this: you will even look more beautiful or more handsome! Now and again you may have seen someone that caught your eye for all the vitality that was seeping out of them. That will be you catching everybody else's eye! Your colouring will be alive, your skin will be glowing, your cells plump with hearty healthiness, your eyes bright. Yes, bright-eyed and bushy tailed! That's you, recharged, rejuvenated and ready to take the world on. Is it ready for you?

Can I do this on my own?

Many find following the plan on their own easier, as that way they have full control of what goes in the fridge without worrying about others' palates. There are fewer temptations when going through this alone, so there are advantages. Yet, some of us need to feel team support or, at least the recognition that we are trying to keep to a plan so that we can be more committed. It depends how disciplined you are. Even if you feel you're not a disciplined type, show yourself otherwise this time. Clean the slate and decide you can be disciplined where things matter, and a good clean out and a rest for your body does matter.

What if my family or partner isn't joining me?

Try and make this work in your favour. Include your partner in your quest and get them enthused rather than feeling isolated. Any kind of self-care, whether that is exercise, diet or meditation can appear to have a selfish side to it, so any sensitivity towards them will help. Remind them that your improved wellbeing makes a difference to your moods, reaction and general feeling of tranquillity within. Don't make it 'your' thing and do your best to keep too much talk about your new habits to yourself. Throughout this programme you'll notice and feel changes that words don't express well enough. Although if we were to find the words, the details of how we feel may not interest our loved ones particularly anyway! So just be positive and let them see what they are getting out of you taking good care of yourself.

Be aware that when we focus on changing our habits that others' habits are highlighted all the more through your eyes and, most likely their own. This doesn't always make people feel very comfortable, so avoid confronting the subject. Maybe they are not ready to change their ways, maybe they don't see reason to or, maybe your healthy habits make them feel out of sorts. They might also be a reminder of the improvements they could be making given the desire or discipline. From some and hopefully very few, there may even be the odd unnecessary remark that could throw you off course. If they are envious, all the better! At least then they will be in the mindset to have some of that good stuff too, and you can show them how. You'll be trimmer, glowing and feeling balanced. Really these are things we should be wishing for each other.

So rise above it. You are feeling better and your change will be good for them. Some might feel they've lost their drinking partner or tea shop friend, but they haven't. It's just that we are entitled to choice and in the meantime your choice is to shape up!

What if you are a busy person?

Get organised. If you're a busy type you'll be used to planning well so that your objectives are achieved. If you're not well organised, don't panic. There is actually no more time required for this plan than your usual meal preparation time **BUT** there is more thinking ahead needed.

One of the biggest steps you'll be making over the next 28 days is a change of habits. Changing habits always feels like the brain is having to re-wire for a bit, so allow for that. There won't be any queuing up at a shop to buy a quick lunch. Instead, that time will be spent eating the lunch your prepared earlier. It is just a matter of jiggling time slots around. Make an extra few minutes in the morning or before going out to put a snack into your bag or make a pack lunch.

Obviously family comes first, but to be able to offer them more we have to be on good form. A grumpy, toxic parent or partner, no matter how efficient, doesn't bring as much to the unit as an upbeat, vitality-filled one. Taking thought, time and care over the next 28 days will ensure you are just that. The extra reserve you'll have for fractious moments in the home will surprise you. One of the most common points people remark on during these weeks, is how level both mood and energy become.

The exercise is a big part of this plan so, no matter your busy timetable, make time for these short sessions. And they are short, you can get a workout done in 12 minutes which, short as it sounds, makes a world of difference. Do what it takes to fit those minutes in. If it means rising 12 minutes earlier to get the morning routine rolling, then do that. Exercising is known to help with clarity and thought process, so remember its value to your day, to this plan and to your ultimate goal.

All the goodness that you'll be feeding yourself with doesn't stop with you looking and feeling good. You will be more alert, have more energy for your work and family and be better equipped to conquer the day's jobs with all that gets thrown at you.

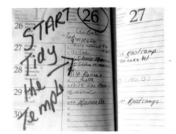

PREPARATION SECTION

So what is the plan for the next 28 days?

We are keeping this simple and easy to follow so there is no room for confusion or error!

How do I get going?

Find a day that suits you to start. Once you have picked the best day for you, you should refer to the daily messages to help you get prepared and motivated. These will start three days before your kick off day. They will guide you in nicely to the days ahead and to the fabulous you that will emerge at the other end … full of vitality and sparkle!

Three days before you start

Take a look at what is coming. Turn to the first shopping list and see what foods you'll need to buy to make things as easy as possible for yourself. Glance through the section 'A Meeting with Myself' on page 43 to give yourself time to work out what you'd like to achieve from this. Also take a look at the exercise section to see what you need to get together for the workouts.

Two days before you start

Take a look at some of the recipes and refer to their shopping lists to help you get ahead on the preparation. Either on this day or the following day, prior to starting you'll need to stock up on a few things. Start clearing out the junk from the larder and cupboards. Get your mind around the process of out with the old and in with the new. Turn to page 44 and read about the importance of an eating journal. Look at the sample one and draw up some of your own.

The day before you start

Make sure you get stocked up. What snacks have you chosen? What is planned for lunch and supper? Being ahead in thought will ensure discipline and success these next couple of days. Get your goals written down, find your measuring tape or string and test the scales. Arrange that you have sufficient water if your tap water isn't so palatable, decide on tomorrow's breakfast, lay out your workout kit and get to bed early. We're leaving adrenaline behind now and a good night's rest is a big part of that.

When to get started

Depending on how your days are timetabled with work and other commitments, you may want to consider starting on a day that will make things flow as easily as possible for you.

It maybe that Monday is a good day for a fresh start for you. Or starting before a weekend may suit better.

Bear in mind that it isn't uncommon for energy levels to be below par for the first few days while the body adjusts to these healthy changes. Also consider there could be other odd discomforts while we purge our mini-addictions – headaches, feeling a little out of sorts etc.

Don't let this postpone your decision by any means and be assured that you can operate perfectly adequately regardless of symptoms. But it is always an idea to try to make a plan that can run smoothly, with as few obstacles as possible.

Everyone is different and therefore symptoms, if any, will vary and fall on different days. From a general observation though, you are most likely to feel the changes on day three. But this is nothing that a good snack (as recommended in the snack section) won't sort out.

How do I prepare?

Take a look at 'Before you start' (page 52) in the daily messages section to set yourself up for success; what to buy, what to throw out and how to record your progress. To make sure this really works for you, you'll find the following information in the 'Getting Going' section (page 42):

- a list of foods that you can choose from
- meal and snack ideas
- an eating journal
- a quick guide to getting started
- 'Before your start' preparation
- 'A Meeting with Myself' page for your motivation

That is all you need to get going.

What will I have to help me?

The lists and tools above will greatly improve your chances of success during the duration of this plan. For instance, the eating journal is for you to log what you've consumed.

From running these courses it is clear to see how some stumble more than others. The exercise in writing down what you eat keeps things focused and honest. It also helps as a reference to look at later. Often in looking back at an eating journal, you can spot small errors that affect things later, whether that be missing a snack, feeling dizzy or fancying starchy foods.

A Meeting with Myself (page 43) is about working out your goals for this plan, getting them on paper and making them real, within days and weeks.

The recipes are a huge help so if you're eating chicken and broccoli every meal, you only have yourself to blame! There are simple, tasty choices and to make things even easier, shopping lists for each meal.

Remember that changing habits and routine requires more thinking and preparation time. What we usually prepare for our meals is quickly done and

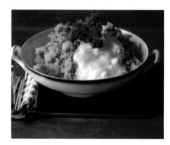

Millet Cauliflower

Nutty Mixed Salad (p29)	Serves 1	2 large lettuce leaves	handful of rocket	¼ pepper	1 radish	4 cherry tomatoes	½ thumb size spring onion	handful cashews, pine nuts, sunflower and poppy seeds	2 brazil nuts
Salad Dressing (p29)	Serves 1	1 tbsp soy sauce	1 small garlic clove	olive oil	sprinkle parsley	1 tsp mustard			
Millet Cauliflower (p30)	Serves 2	150g/5 oz millet	1 tbsp natural veg stock powder	1 small cauliflower head	2 garlic cloves	1 tsp each of ground cumin, paprika, curry powder	handful fresh parsley	1 large red onion	1 dollop natural yoghurt
	60g/2 oz frozen peas								
Stuffed Tomatoes (p31)	Serves 2	2 large, relatively hard beef tomatoes	½ courgette	½ yellow pepper	½ onion	¼ cucumber	1 tbsp lemon juice	1 tbsp coriander	1 tbsp olive oil
		1 tbsp curry powder	1 tbsp cumin seed	250g/9 oz beef mince	1 tbsp natural beef stock powder				

Sample recipe shopping list

achieved without much thought. This plan may feel rather different to your usual habits. Allow for extra time to think through your snacks and meals and prepare them. This way you'll really keep on top of yourself, your planning and therefore results.

In addition just follow your daily messages from 1 to 28, according to the day you are on. These messages will accompany you throughout the process. They are really key to keeping you focused. They will help you understand what is happening, reassure you, guide you and give you tips and support throughout the four weeks. I'm your coach taking you through this, from beginning to end and these messages are my words to you.

The food that you will be eating is simple and nutritious. You can buy all of it from a good supermarket, or butcher's and grocery shop. There are no shakes, meal replacement drinks or snack bars. We're going natural, green and clean. This is the pure and simple approach.

This will mean plenty of vegetables, fruit, vegetable proteins, meat and fish, all of it fresh. If man or manufacturing has spruced it up a bit in any way, leave it alone for now. Just keep to the options provided. The food in the first few days is honest and simple and it may surprise you how much you rely on a splash of this and that to brighten your dishes up. The recipe ideas section will help you to make flavours that will replace bottles and tubes of pastes and sauces.

You may also wonder why some 'healthy' and other natural food choices aren't featured on the list. There is plenty of other food that offers nutritional value as much as those listed, but since we're looking to control cravings and taste buds, and stabilise blood sugar levels, some options are omitted. It isn't because they have been deemed unhealthy for 'tidying the temple', it is just much more effective and easier to eliminate them in the first few days and some, for the whole duration. There is a 'Moving Forward' section that will guide you to reintroducing omitted foods.

Why no potatoes, rice, oats and other grains?

These are all good foods with their own nutritional value. However, if shaping up is your goal then omitting these starchier food types will take you all the way. Cutting down on calories isn't the aim. In fact you won't be counting calories at all.

The aim is to train the body to use its fat reserves to provide you with energy and not to rely on certain food types to deliver energy.

How often will I eat and how much?

You must eat 5 times per day: three meals and two snacks at 2 ½–3 hour intervals. This is vital for the following reasons:

1. to keep and encourage the metabolism to be at good speed
2. to fuel dense tissue (muscle)
3. to reduce the release of insulin activity
4. and therefore, to reduce cravings

There aren't really any limits to quantities other than sensible ones. A general guideline for each meal would be the size of your two hands cupped together and heaped with food, maybe even a bit more in the first days. Snacks would be one handful, say an apple and 10 whole almonds.

Take a look at the sample of a day's food in the **'What will I eat each day?'** paragraph. It is likely that it is more than you eat normally. Do you eat 5 times a day, everyday? Do you eat breakfast plus 2 reasonable meals per day everyday? What many of us do is substitute a meal for a sandwich or other snack type food. It may seem like we're eating a lot with a piece of pie, bread or cake here and there but actually this is empty food. And the more empty food, the hungrier and usually fatter, we get.

What about proportions?

Each dish, meal or snack must have a balance of carbohydrates and proteins. These are listed on page 47 to page 49.

If you were to imagine splitting your plate into three sections, rather like a party taster plate, you would fill one third with protein and the other two thirds with vegetables, or salad, or both.

In the early days you will probably want some more textured food like lentils or chickpeas. Vegetarians may want to make half of their plate protein choices. Ultimately we are looking for a mix of protein and plant, some of it raw. There is more about raw on page 80.

Making do

While fresh is absolutely best, we are aware that some of the recipes have some ingredients that are hard to find fresh or require preparation that may not be ideal for you. For example, chickpeas and red beans are great fillers and add texture to casseroles, burgers and many other dishes. However, preparing them will mean rinsing and then soaking them for a recommended amount of time. Read the labels well. There are tinned options but do look through the ingredients to ensure that you won't be consuming added extras unknowingly.

What will I eat each day?

There are lists of food types on page 47 and 48 that you can choose from and mix together. This first list is just for the first few days. The food is basic and simple – a good choice of vegetables and salads plus all proteins, both vegetarian and meat.

Think of foods that you need to chew, food that your teeth were designed for … to crunch and bite, and take longer to digest for all the right reasons. We are choosing food that the body can assimilate or harmonise with. That is what these days ahead are made up of. The first few days will be especially 'clean'. You won't go hungry, but you might think that you are hungry. That is the feeling that you will soon be able to identify as a craving rather than hunger. There's a difference!

A TYPICAL SAMPLE OF A DAY'S EATING

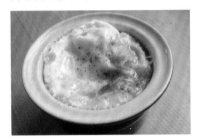

Breakfast *Fresh fruit followed by an egg.*

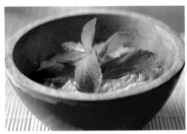

Snack *Crudités (handful of chopped vegetables, carrots, cucumber etc.) and homemade houmous dip (chick-peas) or slices of tempeh.*

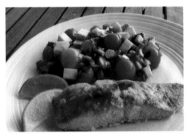

Lunch *A fish steak, a salad with steamed or raw vegetables added for bulk. Maybe lentils to add volume to the meal.*

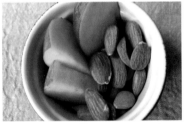

Snack *A piece of fruit, e.g. an apple and a small handful of almonds.*

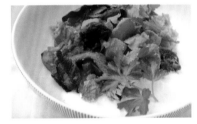

Supper *A soup from the recipe section followed by a casserole of meat or vegetarian protein alternative and plenty of vegetables or salad.*

REMEMBER

To drink a mix of water, freshly juiced juices from fruit and vegetables, and herbal teas.

What won't I be eating?

Processed foods, refined foods, caffeine and toxins.

There are some fruits you won't be eating either. That is because some are higher in fructose and turn to glycogen quickly, resulting in storing energy that we don't want stored. You will eat flours and grains towards the end of the plan but only whole grain ones.

Think of all those soft foods that you barely need to chew, such as muffins, pastas, breads and crisps. These are of little nutritional value. Consider them dead as far as offering you anything other than a few minutes of fun.

About the stages of the plan

Days 1–4

The first 4 days are effectively the detox time. It is during this stage we are trying to get on top of cravings. It is the most likely time that you will have cravings but, once you have three days of clean eating behind you, you'll be well away.

Will I have lost weight by now?

It is usual for many in the first few days that waistbands become looser. For some this will be any previous bloating or water retention subsiding, while the body's cells return to their healthy chemical balance. For others, it is the start of an effective fat loss period. This period is designed to mobilise fat efficiently, which is why there are no starchy or sugary foods.

Fat loss is a slower procedure than many weight loss plans will admit to. To lose 10lbs in 10 days for instance can be possible. We all know that from sickness or other malnourished moments. BUT is that 10lbs of fat? No, it would be a mix of water, muscle and lastly, fat. To ensure this weight doesn't return days after finishing the plan, we want to be sure that it is *only* fat and water retention that goes.

Keeping the metabolism efficient is key to this plan. We do that by regular eating. Eating less, or less frequently, causes the metabolism to slow down, it goes into a 'conserving fuel' mode (of storing our fat and stored sugars) for an impending crisis of starvation. You may have noticed after a period of sickness and being bed-bound you come out skinnier BUT your muscles are empty, this is when your body has flushed out excess water and within days, the weight is back on you.

Given the right care the body will burn fat for fuel, otherwise its tendency is to slow the metabolism and maintain the fat. Like a fire, we have to keep stoking it and feeding it to keep it burning. Keeping your eating levels high and making up for lost carbohydrates such as rice, potatoes, cereals etc. means compensating with a high vegetable and salad intake.

How often should I be doing my workouts?

The first week we're aiming for every other day. This gives the muscles time to recover and, while the body makes adjustments at this early stage of the plan, it is possible that you may not feel energised enough to push through exercise sessions daily. But the exercise sessions are short, so if you feel you can exercise everyday, do. If you've been used to resistance training and pushing weights, then go for it and exercise daily. Although be sure to take one day's rest in the week.

How much will my exercise routine help during this stage?

Greatly. As we're stressing, we're looking to speed up the metabolism. Bursts of energy, especially as designed in our fitness section, will deliver this. Not just for the moments that you're doing your workout, but for as long as 24 hours afterwards. Luckily for many of us, short bursts of more intensive exercise, combined with resistance moves or pushing weights, brings exactly what we're seeking – better fitness, improved muscular tone and an efficient metabolism along with fat loss. All achieved without taking too much out of our day.

Will I get bulky muscles?

No. An important side to this plan is building or at least maintaining good muscle condition. Having good muscle density serves for many reasons but in our case it is key for shedding extra fat long-term. We're looking to feed the muscles, starve the fat and get the body working efficiently. Just a little more muscle tone raises the metabolism. That means even if you're having an inactive day, you'll still be burning more energy than if you were out of shape with less muscle tone having an inactive day.

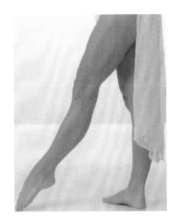

If bulking up and becoming Miss Universe is a concern for you, forget that worry for now. It is very hard to build a lot of muscle, not to mention quickly. You'd have to be entirely dedicated to add on the kilos of muscle. The exercises and eating plan during these days are for creating condition, tone, good shape, strength (mental and physical!) and for feeling a lot fitter.

How will I be feeling?

It is during this time that you may suffer withdrawal symptoms or simply feel a bit different. Many people feel mental clarity at this stage, sleep is normally improved and despite a lack of zest from the muscles themselves, patchy spells of day time tiredness may have gone. But come evening, you may be ready for an early night.

There is a lot of change going on during this time. Allow the body rest while it accommodates the changes. For those who are used to whizzing about and running on adrenaline there may be some reactions and strong signs that the adrenals need a rest.

REMEMBER

So long as you keep eating regularly from the foods on the list and make time for a good night's sleep, you'll cope very well. A few more food choices come in by Day 4.

More information The early days of the plan

Often around day three, some people feel a little 'empty'. Not hungry, but as if they need to fuel up, rather as if the tank is running low and getting to the top of the stairs is more of an ordeal!

Trust that you are just going through changes and that it will pass. Mostly people get past this feeling by day five or six, some within a day.

However it is more noticeable with more active types. It drags on a bit longer for them. It could be that their demands are too high while the body is trying to make adjustment so it is therefore an indicator to slow down. Or, it could be that they are just a little more in tune with their energy levels.

If slowing down is not an option, and it often isn't for people involved in sports or physical labour, hold tight and be assured that it just takes a few days longer. It will be worth it.

Days 5–10

How will I be feeling?

By now most of the symptoms could have passed but don't worry if they haven't, your body is just being very thorough in its clearing out. Energy levels should be picking up and soon surpassing what they used to be, especially throughout the day. You may feel more even-tempered and more on top of things.

There may be the odd craving but abstain all you can, being led into temptation will upset the calm waters you've created and makes for a bumpier ride later. By that I mean it is easier to not cheat than to cheat because the choice of food or drink may not only upset the blood sugar levels, but give you a taste for more. This makes it harder to get back on track and keep cravings at bay. It takes longer than these few days to change habits naturally so give it your commitment, you'll be pleased you did.

You'll have the energy for daily workouts now. They only take a few minutes so just do them. There is no need to lose time getting ready. Just wear easy-to-move -in clothes and a pair of trainers. Ladies will need a good supportive bra. Your muscles will be used to the moves so there should be no more aching this week … well maybe a little as we pick up the pace!

Is there more food to add?

Yes, at this stage we broaden the fruit choices, add some other things that will help flavour dishes and add some live culture into the intestines.

Things will be picking up now, you'll be in the mode for progress and you'll realise that you feel good on this plan. You'll feel nourished and clean! Weight loss during this period maybe slower but it isn't the end of change and all things good. Plenty more of that to come! External changes may be less obvious during this time but change comes from the inside first.

Days 11–22

It is at this stage that we can introduce some complex carbohydrates. If you have been really missing them, here's your chance to get your teeth into the texture of some of the grains and cereal listed.

If by this stage you're not missing the bulk that carbohydrates bring, maybe hold out a little longer. We're still in the interim stages of the plan and you'll be used to the new you – bad eating habits behind you, eating regularly, fuelling well and not least, stable blood sugar levels. So you may be taking these for granted now and wondering what's next?

As the daily messages will inform you, true fat loss and allowing the organs to detox, takes time. When you bear in mind the months or years we spend making ourselves toxic, there needs to be a reasonable chance in time of undoing that. In fairness, the body does this incredibly quickly and efficiently for all the abuse, but

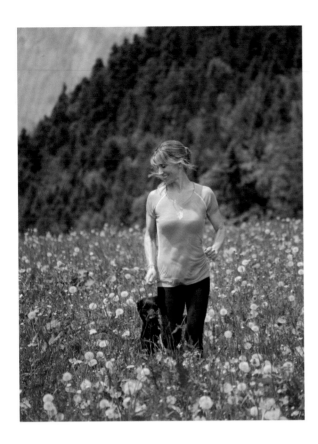

it can't do it over night. We want good results and long-term ones. Bear in mind that while you are fuelling your body with health and wholesome things, it is quietly doing its best repair job possible. Be kind and patient to you and your body!

The last six days

It is around this time that you'll be changing your habits for the long-term. We need this long to form new habits and if you've kept to the plan you'll really be ready to resist your usual temptations for quite a time yet. Fat loss may well pick up again during this time but if it doesn't, trust that it will within time. Condition will still be improving and you will be quite used to your clearer skin and less water retention. Rather like a child growing up, there are stages during this plan when we see no progress but there is always something progressing. For example, an infant may stop growing while his teeth are breaking through. For us, fat loss could slow down while other more important changes are occurring.

More food is added and you'll be learning to expand your cuisine within these choices. This will broaden your nutritional intake which is important for the healthy balance we're looking for. To omit list five's final food options long-term would be compromising on good and easily available nutrients. So be sure to add them in.

GETTING GOING
The Quick Start Guide

During this four week plan you will shape up, lose fat, increase your energy levels, get fitter, have more vitality, ditch the bad moods and get the very best out of your health and self. You will not just feel great, you will also … LOOK GREAT! And, you will get plenty of compliments. Whatever your shape or size you are going to see results here.

There are lots of things to get going with so get familiar with the points below:

- read the 'Meeting with Myself' on page 43 and write down your goals
- copy out what you need to buy in from the shopping list
- refer to the first section of recipes for tasty, quick ideas and shopping needs
- add ideas for your snacks to the shopping list
- read the points on keeping an eating journal on page 44
- weigh and measure yourself and log the details on page 51
- go to the 'Try These Tests' on page 30 and make notes on your condition
- take photos (see page 51)

Then start reading the daily messages and dig deep to find 100% commitment for the next 28 days. Read a message for each day, according to the day you are on. They are there to encourage you, so lap them up. Apart from much more explanation and information, there may be parts in these messages that strike a chord with you and help keep you all the more motivated.

Other points to consider

The first few days will require the most discipline. When you've got those behind you, you'll be thrilled to start feeling and seeing the changes.

There are some great ideas for meals in the recipe section. But you could also get your own cook books out and modify the recipes to suit the food list.

There is so much to learn about food and nutrition over these weeks. Not textbook learning, but living and feeling the differences.

Make this your best chance ever to getting the best out of yourself!

A Meeting with Myself

Take a moment to think about what you would like to get out of these next four weeks. What ultimately do you want to see from yourself during this time, and beyond?

Break it into three or four goals. Make sure they really mean something to you and the thought of them leaves you feeling uplifted.

Write them down somewhere you can refer to them often. Be specific with your wording and write them down as if you have already achieved them, e.g. I feel much better … my legs are slimmer … I'm in control of my habits … I am a dress size smaller … I am taking care of myself … my moods are even … etc. Whatever it is for you that lifts your spirits, note it down.

Spend a moment picturing your goals and targets.

Now take it a stage further …

Take a moment to go through the following:

Imagine you have a very important meeting to prepare for. It needs to be clear in your mind and it needs an agenda, especially since you are the director. Keep imagining. To help you out with the meeting, you can delegate points to others. Only these 'others' are just duplicates of you. One big meeting with lots of 'yous'. Each of them sitting in front of you have a role in what you are going to achieve in the days ahead. Below are some ideas of the roles each 'you' could perform.

To *Tidy the Temple* and glow from within, these elements need to be thought through in the days ahead:

- organisation and preparation
- discipline and focus
- health and fitness
- general balance of the day, rest, fun, work and self care

Now, for each one of these points exampled above, ask yourself:

- where am I at now with this?
- what do I need to do to improve on this?
- what are the steps I need to take?
- what does the end result look like?

Go through these slowly. Then make some notes that identify some actions you may need to take. (See page 76 for an example).

Keep these notes and look at them regularly to make sure you are up to speed.
Meeting over!

My goals

* *I am sleeping well +
  my body is regenerating
  + rejuvenating*

* *I am slimmer with
  toned muscles and
  fresher, younger skin*

* *I have much more
  vitality, energy and
  mental clarity*

Key to success

All sorts of research on how to achieve goals, stresses the importance of writing the goals down. Other props, mental images and auditory help (like affirmations) also have their value so if things like this appeal to you, get creating.

REMEMBER

Come back to this meeting with yourself whenever you wish to renew your goals. Bringing your imagination into it makes it more vivid, more fun and prints your desires firmly in your mind.

It also adds structure and confidence to your journey to a healthier and brighter you.

PERSONAL POINT

On one of my courses I made the mistake of not emphasising how important it was for the participants to write down their goals. Instead I gave it as an option.

It was foolish as I'd made the decision the team was all grown up and probably fed up of being told what to do. My error was quickly evident. Individuals' momentum slipped and at some points, many of us forgot all the good reasons why we wanted to do this clean up. Although we got through it successfully, it was made harder by the lack of clarity of our ultimate goals.

The thing is, however adult and responsible we are, being told what to do is exactly what we need, to see something through effectively. Even when I'm 'tidying the temple' on my own, I always stir up some inspiration and write my goals down.

Eating Journal

Keeping a record of what you eat and when you eat it may seem like extra work and not a priority, but it is vital to success. Plenty of experiments prove how effective it is to note down food and eating patterns for both discipline and achievement's sake.

Experiments aside, from experience with groups, those who record these points stay on track and complete their tidying up thoroughly.

So read on and help yourself by keeping an eating journal:

- maintaining an honest and accurate journal of everything you eat and drink is key to your fat loss success. On the eating journal page, note the day, the times you eat, how you feel just before eating (tired, stressed, anxious, excited etc.) and how you felt about an hour after eating.

- with the use of the notes you will be able to track patterns that you have built up over time without realising. Drops of energy, moods and food cravings will be indicative of these patterns.

- keeping an eye on your food consumption and choices will also help you understand why fat loss may be stalling.

- these records will be an excellent future reference when comparing your condition and habits of then, to now.

- make a note of who you eat with or the environment that encourages those food choices.

- it takes 3 minutes to do, so ensure you take your time to fill in the diary each day.

Logging your food intake is CRUCIAL to the success of the plan.

REMEMBER

Use this food log to keep on top of your goals. Make further copies to see you through the duration.

FOOD LOG

Day	Time	How was your mood or energy before eating?	What did you eat?	How much did you eat? light/medium/large portion	How was your mood or energy after eating?	Where were you and who joined you?	Notes

Food lists

The food lists are based around reducing cravings, mobilising fat, clearing out toxicity and revving up the metabolism. Many other benefits come as a result of this.

Why no grains, oats, brown rice or quinoa in the early stages? These are great foods but at this stage we're also looking to mobilise fat and fuel our muscles. We want the body to draw on resources other than our stored carbohydrate and blood sugar.

NOTE: If you're used to 60–70 % of the food on your plate being carbohydrates (pasta, rice, sandwiches, croissants and any other starchy food) there will be a massive deficit in calories. Considerably less calories than you are used to could backfire causing your metabolism to slow down. Alongside that, there may be a loss of lean tissue which we want to keep. To get round that problem make sure you make up for the loss of carbohydrate calories and eat plenty of lighter proteins and vegetables.

It won't matter that you may be eating more than before. These foods will assimilate well with your body and that is what matters.

Processed foods and anything with E numbers in must GO! If you don't understand the ingredients don't buy it. If it has been cut and cooked it is fair to say it will have ingredients in that we need to eliminate for the first few days.

If it doesn't grow, don't buy it. Not for now.

Ratios and portions

Your plate needs a good balance of fibre and protein. Ensure that at least two thirds of the plate is salad and/or vegetables, or even fruit. The other third is protein. Keep this ratio the same for snacks. If you are a vegetarian you may need a half and half mix of vegetable protein and fibre. The same ratio will be good for snacks.

Don't concern yourself with portions for the first few days, it is the quality of food that matters now. It is much more beneficial to eat a full plate of food than not enough. Once you have settled into the new habits you may want a clearer idea as to how much you should be eating.

- **A tasty tip:** Chop up a clump of your chosen herb, mix with some oil and ground nuts, season with salt and pepper, then sprinkle over meat, fish or vegetables to add some great flavour.
- For a basic chicken and vegetable stock recipe see page 57.
- Seasoning (sea salt and pepper) can be used freely.

List 1 *Food from Day 1*

PROTEINS: One to be eaten every meal

■ *HEAVIER PROTEINS* ■ *VEGETARIAN OPTIONS*

Cod	Crab	Haddock	Lobster	Mackerel
Monkfish	Prawns	Salmon	Sardines	Sea Bass
Shellfish	Sole	Swordfish	Tuna	
Beef	Chicken	Duck	Kidney	Lamb
Parma ham (with no added preservatives)	Pork	Turkey	Veal	All nuts
Chickpeas (tinned if necessary)	Eggs	Hemp seed	Houmous	Lentils
Seeds	Soya *(in moderation)*	Tempeh (fermented soybeans)		

■ Depending where you live, ostrich, game and horse meats may be an option. Consider these latter two to be heavy proteins.

■ Abstain from cow's milk and other dairy products during the 28 days, except organic, live natural yoghurt which is best kept to a minimum.

FRUIT

Apples	Grapefruit	Lemons	Limes	Melon
Olives	Oranges	Pears	Pomegranates	

SALADS AND VEGETABLES

All leafy greens	All types of squash	Artichoke	Asparagus	Avocado
Aubergine	Broccoli	Cabbage (green and red)	Carrots	Cauliflower
Celery	Courgette	Cucumber	Fennel	*Fresh herbs:* parsley, basil, mint, sage, thyme etc.
Garlic	Ginger	Green beans	Kale	Leek
Mushroom	Onion and spring onion	Parsnip	Peas	Raw mung bean sprouts and all germinating seeds
Red and yellow pepper	Rocket	Seaweed	Spinach	Tomatoes

List 1 *Food from Day 1 continued overleaf*

OILS

Almond oil	Coconut oil	Flax oil	Hemp oil	Olive oil
Peanut oil	Sesame oil	Walnut oil		

- When oil is heated, the composition and molecules change for the worse. Coconut oil is an exception and can be heated up to 170 degrees without any detrimental changes. Try to avoid overheating oils.

DRINKS

Coconut water	Freshly squeezed juice, homemade juices and smoothies (p14 of recipe section)	Fruit tea	Green tea	Herbal tea
Water				

List 2 *Food to introduce on Day 4*

FRUIT

Blueberries	Peaches	Pineapple	Raspberries	Strawberries

OTHER

All legumes, white and red kidney Beans	All spices and dry herbs	All pulses	Balsamic and apple cider vinegar	Live organic cow, sheep or goat yoghurt

List 3 *Food to introduce on Day 11*

FRUIT

Apricots	Blackberries	Blackcurrants	Cherries	Cranberries
Grapes	Plums	Redcurrants		

SALAD AND VEGETABLES

Beetroot	Radishes

GRAINS

Barley	Buckwheat	Millet	Oats

OTHER

Crunchy flaked soya (in moderation)	Smoked fish (e.g. salmon, mackerel)	Soy sauce (all natural ingredients)	Rice, oat, spelt and almond milk in moderation

List 4 *Food to introduce on Day 21*

FRUIT

Fresh figs

OTHER

Coconut	Coconut milk (natural)	Stock: if you prefer to buy stock, use one with all natural ingredients

List 5 *Food to introduce on Day 26*

GRAINS

Brown rice	Quinoa	Rye	Spelt

FLOURS

Barley	Buckwheat	Chestnut	Corn
Millet	Oat	Rye	Spelt

OTHER

Peanut/nut butter (all natural without hydrogenated fat)	Pumpernickel bread	Rye bread	Slow-acting yeast

Some fruits have more fructose than others, some taste sweeter and some have a higher glycemic index. Depending on an eating plan's approach, these factors and fruit choices, will vary in favour and may be confusing to the health conscious individual. Overall, eating more fruit in its fresh and raw state is always going to be much more beneficial than cooked, processed, pre-packaged or very acidic food. Tidy the Temple's goal is to tame the taste buds and so the majority of sweeter and softer fruits are introduced over time.

In List 3, to be introduced on Day 11, there are the following grains that can be introduced: Barley, buckwheat, oat and millet. By Day 26 and List 5, grains and flours feature more. Use these sparingly to avoid ending up in a carbohydrate heavy and over acidic eating plan. Try rotating carbohydrates and omitting on alternate days as suggested in daily message 11 and on page 147.

Your Vital Statistics!

PERSONAL POINT

From years of measuring body fat percentages with reliable equipment, it is obvious that during the first week of people doing more exercise and improving their eating habits, that the changes in fat percentage are very marginal. Don't be discouraged by this.

As mentioned before, fat is slow to mobilise, it isn't like water and muscle that makes a big drop or difference on the weighing scales.

But realise that losing as little as 2% fat, minimal as that sounds, is actually a significant amount of fat weight, this could be a few kilos or some pounds of pure fat.

Taking a fat reading at the start and end of the 28 days shows the efficacy of the plan and is much more encouraging than weekly readings.

About measuring yourself

Making notes of your measurements before, during and after the next few weeks is another crucial part to success. The scales may vary but your measurements remain true. Many ladies have been through stages of the course worrying with the likes of 'I haven't lost any weight this week but my clothes are looser'. Weight isn't really an issue, but what your weight is made up of is. For many of us, how we look and feel in our clothes matters; so it is your body size, shape and measurements that are of more relevance than your weight.

Fat measuring devices

There are a few other ways that you can measure your body and that is by measuring its composition i.e. how much fat, water and muscle you are made up of. Some weighing scales these days have this option. Have a look in the information box on page 51 to find out more about these.

Measure yourself

- Around the chest at nipple level
- Around the waist at tummy button level
- Around the hips at the largest part
- *In addition, you may also like to measure your legs and arms*
- For the legs, wrap the measuring tape around the top of the leg just where the fold of the buttock on the back of the leg sits. Measure both legs.
- For the arms, measure the length of your upper arm from shoulder to a bent elbow. Say this is 30 cm, find half way at 15 cm and measure around the arm. Make sure you do both arms.

Note the figures in the Weight and Measurements Log box on page 51, or somewhere that you refer to often, e.g. your diary. If you can't dig out a tape measure use a dressing gown tie or a belt and use safety pins to mark your measurement.

Weigh yourself

Check your scales are in working order. If they are not, check that they are consistent with their readings. Even if you don't like what they say, note the reading down and make sure that every time you weigh yourself again, that the scales are in the same place and on the same surface as before. With some scales, readings can vary from hard to soft surfaces.

WEIGHT AND MEASUREMENTS LOG

	WEIGHT	WAIST	HIPS	CHEST	ARMS	LEGS
Start						
Day 7						
Day 14						
Day 21						
Day 28						

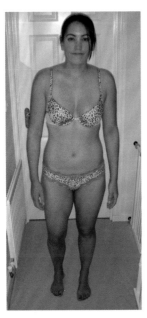
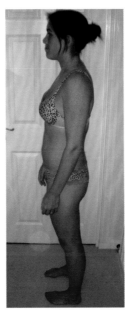
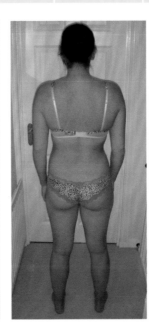

Take three photos

- One of you facing the camera

- One side shot

- One with your back to the camera

Note where you stood and your camera position. This will make for the best comparisons afterwards. This is worthwhile as it will be a good reminder of how much change you can make during this time and will motivate you for another time.

More information Specialist fat-measuring devices

These can vary in quality, accuracy and reading depending on a few things like when you last ate, if you've just had a coffee or if you've just been very active.

If the device is for standing on, as if you would with regular weighing scales, you may find that you get a rather generous reading and it says that you hold more fat than you do.

This is because the reading and electrodes' connectivity only passes through both legs and the backside. It can't read the entire body.

So if you carry much of your weight around those areas and little on your upper body, it would register your fattiest part and make a disappointing and incorrect reading. Likewise is the case with apparatus

that you may just hold in your hands. It would only read your upper body's fat.

More accurate are apparatus for which you need to lie down and have electrodes attached to your hand and foot. Correct and informative as they are, they are pricey but you may find a fitness club or trainer will offer this service. They may even have the facilities to work out your body composition by measuring you in a pool. Another possibility is the original 'fat calliper' method which is literally a calliper that pinches and measures fat.

More importantly, above the accuracy of the device, is that you use the same device each time you weigh and measure yourself, no matter the technique or technology.

DAILY MESSAGES

To keep you motivated and interested

Before you start

You've decided you're going to commit the next four weeks to really turning your health and shape around. Well done!

So that you are well prepared to achieve your goals, there are lots of things to take into consideration. All the tips, support and guidance will be in these daily messages for you.

Make sure you read the preparation section and early messages before launching straight into day one.

You'll also need to measure and weigh yourself, so make sure you have scales and a tape measure. Refer to page 50 for more measuring tips. Remember, if you don't have a measuring tape you can use cord or a soft belt and place a safety pin for the measurement point.

Now is a good time to clear out the junk foods from your larder, life and liver. So go through the cupboards, tins and 'stash' places and get rid of anything that may be of temptation. Give it to someone else or any other options that come to mind, just clear it out and away. If it is there, you'll eat it. If it isn't there, you'll go for the healthy option every time. Make room for success now.

Take a look at the first food list (page 47).

Make sure you find the time to buy your choice of produce from the list. Most things are available from a good supermarket but, for instance, hemp and coconut oil will need a visit to the local health shop.

Give this 100% commitment.
See how much you can get out of that body of yours.

*"As an ex-fitness model and competitor, I know all about pulling all the stops out and having to shape up sensibly for lasting results.
Whatever our shape or size, we are going to see results here."*

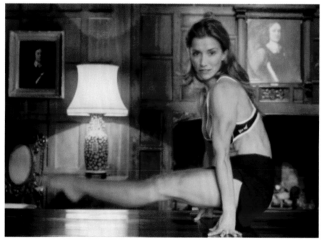

Photo: Nigel Harper

The day before starting

Tomorrow you'll be on day one of Tidying your Temple!

Sleep well tonight! The next few days may be a little uncomfortable while your body clears out. Headaches, irritability and other symptoms may happen – PLEASE sit them out and let your body re-balance. See it as all the toxins surfacing. It can make you realise how addicted we've become to such things as caffeine, sugar and refined foods.

It will be worth it, I promise!

Take a photo of yourself

Take shots facing the camera, with your back to the camera and a profile shot too. Make sure you note the place where you stood and where the cameraman or self photo was positioned, this makes for real comparisons later with the 'after' photo. Ideally remember the lighting situation, the time of day and whether it was natural lighting or not and match it all as much as you can for next time. Some people skip this part and have only ever regretted it afterwards. Seeing the difference objectively is very motivating and interesting. The changes start early on so get those photos taken before day one.

Take your vital statistics!

Measure and weigh yourself. See page 50 for more information on this.

Be prepared … have enough food!

Preparation is the key to this. That way you have good control of your blood sugar levels. All that stands for steady energy and, as already mentioned, it also eases cravings immensely.

To get the results, we're going to eat **5 times a day.** Forget the 'no-snack-between -meals' rule.

For this we need three decent meals per day **plus** two snacks.

Eat protein with every meal and snack

Select these from the list of proteins on page 47.

Snacks still need to be a combination of something from our fruits, salads and vegetables list and something from the protein list. To keep it simple I'd suggest things like:

- carrots/celery/avocado + tempeh + houmous or a few nuts

OR

- fruit + a few nuts or a protein from the list, even a slice of chicken.

There are more options in the recipe section, page 61.

Exercise

Make sure you have eaten no later than two hours before doing your exercise session. If you plan to work out first thing in the morning and eating that much beforehand is impractical, eat breakfast post-exercise. Just make sure you do that workout very soon after getting up. Avoid putting it off and therefore delaying eating. Blood sugar levels will drop and it will be a bad and disadvantageous start to the day. You could always opt for a piece of fruit 45 minutes before starting the session.

After exercising, eat a snack if you've had a good breakfast or make up a good breakfast straight after if you didn't have one. All these small courses of actions help prevent fancying a nice cake later on in the day!

Ideas for breakfast tomorrow

Breakfast needs more thought than other meals so you could try:

- grapefruit with almonds sprinkled on top
- half a melon with seeds and almonds
- scrambled eggs and tomatoes, spinach, onions, etc.
- spinach and mushroom omelettes
- fruit salad with hemp/ground almonds/seeds + a boiled egg

Or you can try combinations of these. Just make sure you get protein and some vegetable and/or fruit. If you're a non-nut eater and don't like eggs, maybe take fruit and slices of tempeh or one of the other proteins. You could even boil up lentils or chickpeas tonight and be well prepared. See pages 14 to 17 in the recipe section for more ideas.

Plan ahead for your meals for tomorrow

- If you are out all day, prepare your vegetables and grill chicken or turkey and take it with you. Maybe steam or cook them as you eat breakfast.
- Prepare your snack box too – pear/apple and a few nuts (unsalted) or raw vegetables and houmous are quick and easy options. See page 61 in the recipe section.
- Don't run out of food! Be prepared and EAT EVERY THREE HOURS.
- For your meals and cooking, go for variety. Use herbs, onions … anything that adds to the taste. Spend the extra few minutes chopping up these extras. It is worth it and keeps the plan more interesting.
- If a food isn't on the shopping list then don't eat it at this time.
- If you find yourself in a restaurant choose well, according to the food list and ratios (on pages 46 and 47). Omit any of the extra sauces.

This is phase one of the plan. Think of this as a detox and a really good cleanse!

Day 1

Take in all the support and tips to make the best success of cleaning up

So think of this … chew! 30 times if you're counting. 'Conscious eating' as it is known. Just eat. No reading while chewing or doing other jobs. Just focus on eating, chewing, placing your knife and fork down and finishing your mouthful before starting again. If you couldn't see what was on your plate then you would use your natural appetite guides much more. Your brain would automatically register when you'd eaten enough and stop!

Chewing and eating in a more controlled way also means your brain has time to give you signals that you don't have time to recognise, such as 'that's enough eating now!'

If you were told to 'finish your plate up' as a youngster, it maybe what you do now, no matter how full you are. You could try eating with a blindfold and see if you finish your plate or not. I'd like a photo of that for my next book if you do! Stop when you've had enough, then take off the blindfold and see how much you have left.

Get going with exercise today. Turn to page 91. Pick your appropriate level, give yourself 13 minutes, turn the music on and get going. No need for fancy workout kit, just get some training shoes on or use bare feet on a soft carpet or mat. The important thing is to move and stir up that metabolism.

To assist the body's water balance, just add a couple of grains of sea salt to 1.5 litres of water. This'll help your body's hydration where it needs it, yet assist in draining the bloating from your cells, which gives us that feeling of holding water. If the water tastes at all salty you've added too much.

Have you weighed and measured yourself and taken the photos? You need to do this for future reference and to see how you started out and how far you've come. And you will be pleased you have. Do this now as in a few days you'll already be looking better!

Keep your goals to hand and present in your thoughts. If you have not written them down, take a moment do so now.

If you are going out, be prepared and take a snack box and water.

Just think, day one of cleaning up. Give it your best shot and start changing habits now.

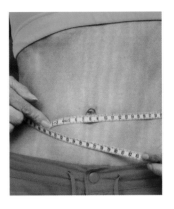

Get prepared

Have you weighed and measured yourself, and taken the photos? You need to do this for future reference and to see how you started out and how far you've come. And you will be pleased you have. Do this now as in a few days you'll already be looking better!

REMEMBER

- Keep to the food on the list
- Keep to the plan
- Write down what you've eaten in your eating journal
- Eat three meals and two snacks
- Eat often, every 2–3 hours, hunger isn't a part of this plan!
- Have a protein portion with each of these (for how much, see page 47)
- Drink water, 1.5 litres throughout the day

Day 2

How did your first day go?
How are your muscles after yesterday's workout?
Did you pick the right level for your current fitness?

If you didn't get that workout in yesterday be sure to do it today, and soon!

Have you taken a photo and/or measured yourself? If not, do it now! Very soon there will be changes and it is good to know what your true starting point was.

Maybe you felt tired by the end of yesterday. That is quite usual. Because there are fewer foods to spark up adrenaline, tiredness can be expected but see it as a good thing.

How about cravings? Just ask yourself, can I possibly be hungry or is this a craving? If you keep to 3 meals and 2 snacks per day, with plenty of vegetables and fruit for volume, it has to be a craving.

Keep drinking water even if it means lots of visits to the lavatory. It is likely that you will urinate more and longer for these first few days, especially if your cells have been holding water. Limit your water consumption to 1.5 to 2 litres per day.

If you do get the odd symptom of withdrawal, a headache, aching joints or even the shakes, **be brave**. Take the hit and let it happen without the help of painkillers.

Make sure you're getting your vegetables and fruit. Courgettes, aubergine and grapefruit are good for filling up on.

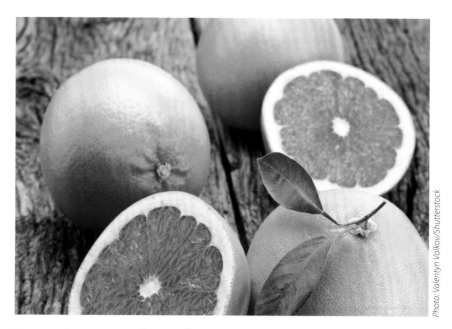

Photo: Valentyn Volkov/Shutterstock

Remember we are doing this to serve a purpose.
Note what you've eaten in the eating journal and keep your goals forefront in your mind.

Make your own stock

This will expand your cuisine.

Having some stock on the side makes all the difference to meals at this stage.

For a chicken stock. Just boil up the bones and carcass in enough water to cover half of it. Throw in a few fresh herbs if you have some, along with sea salt and pepper. Leave it for at least 30 minutes simmering. Pour the fluid through a colander, leave it to cool and store in the fridge. Throw or compost the rest.

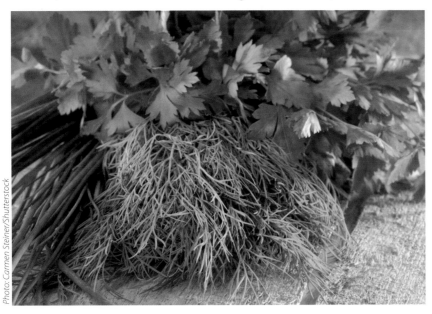

Photo: Carmen Steiner/Shutterstock

For a vegetable stock. Use what you've got – this might be carrot tops, celery tops, the odd stray mushroom, herbs, anything that you don't mind boiling up for flavour alone. Save your fresh produce for eating.

Add a chopped up onion, sea salt and pepper. Cover it well with water, boil up and leave to simmer for at least 30 minutes. Strain, allow the fluid to cool and store in the fridge.

Build your store up and keep the vegetables in freezer bags in the freezer until you need them! Think about also freezing stock in ice cube trays if you just want to add a little bit of flavour to a dish.

At this stage you can thicken the stock to make a sauce. Try ground almonds, boiled pumpkin or carrots, and blend well. You could also use extracted juice pulp.

Day 3

You have made it to Day 3!

So, how is it going so far? Are you still craving things? Any headaches? Or do you feel a bit shaky?

If there is a moment when you feel a little shaky, it will be the withdrawal from relying on certain food types for energy. You're going through a change of energy systems!

The stock of sugar in the blood is reducing and so the body will start drawing from the fat cells. For some there is a noticeable change of energy over this time. So long as you are consuming enough of the vegetable and fruit options, this need not be a concern and will soon pass.

Keep up with your new good habits!

Forget about topping up this void or lack of energy with old habits! Is a bowl of cereal or a piece of bread or chocolate going to fix the problem? No! Let your body see it through. Your new habits aren't poisonous but your body got used to your old ones and has become addicted to these highs of instant and processed food. Now you're feeling the withdrawal.

You may have escaped any suffering! It is usually giving up the caffeine that makes this stage uncomfortable.

If you don't look so great, a bit greyish in skin, be sure to load up well on the foods from the non-protein list. If your bowel movement has slowed down, increase your water intake and likewise make up for lost carbohydrate calories from the vegetables. You could also try relaxing!

Charging around raises adrenal levels and can, for some, slow down going to the lavatory. Another tip you could try is raising your feet on a little step as you're seated on the lavatory.

There are lots of adjustments going on inside you just now so it is inevitable you will feel them.

Take a look at the goals you wrote down. As previously mentioned, it is known that writing goals down (and looking at them again!), and being clear about them, brings 100% more likelihood of you realising them.

My goals
* *I am sleeping well and my body is regenerating and rejuvenating*
* *I am slimmer with toned muscles and fresher, younger skin*
* *I have much more vitality, energy and mental clarity*

Remember your eating journal

Keeping note of the food you've eaten also multiplies your chances of success.

Day	Time	How was your mood or energy before eating?	What did you eat?	How much did you eat? light/medium/large portion	How was your mood or energy after eating?	Where were you and who joined you?	Notes
1	8am	Hungry!	2 grapefruit halves sprinkled with ground almonds	Light	Positive	On my own	Not as hungry as I thought I would be
1	10.30am	Fab!	Handful of cashews and an apple	Medium	Hungry. I ate another handful of cashews and a pear	With my colleagues	Good after my second snack

Keep exercising

There needs to be another exercise session today. If it felt right, go back to the same choice as day one. Soon you'll get familiar with the moves and be able to knock out these sessions fast and effectively.

You may find that energy levels are not on your side but just push that aside and carry on! The workout is short and it'll be over in no time.

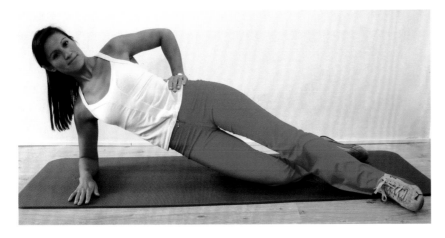

You are committed now so keep going and give it everything!

It isn't long in the scheme of things and results are just around the corner.

Your protein intake

Does it feel like too much protein? It may be just now while you're settling into new habits. Be wary of consuming too much animal protein and remember your vegetable protein choices. Also, if as little as 10% of your meal is protein, it will still trigger a message to the brain saying you're not hungry. So you could cut down on quantity if you fill up well on vegetables and more.

Keep really strong these few days. Eat according to your notes and food list with no additions! Tomorrow you can add more food to add to your list. Take a look at some of the recipes in the cooking section to help you with ideas and help you add some taste into these first days.

Day 4

Already by day four we start to look clearer, even if we're not thinking clearly.

Maybe you're feeling a little giddy, but you're still on track. Well done! Hopefully your muscles feel fine or even a little 'used' from yesterday's workout. So remember … chew, as much as 30 times. Well, some foods such as soft fruits need half that amount. You could try eating with a blindfold as mentioned in Day 1. Why? Well, in tests, if we can't see what we are eating, we tend to eat what we need rather than what we see in front of us.

How does the eating journal look? Keep it updated.

We are now looking at improving the gut's bacterial balance. So, as you can see, yoghurt is now on the menu. There are other foods that contain natural probiotics (good bacteria) but are mainly fermented. For now you may want to keep it simple and choose a good natural live yoghurt or Kefir. Leeks are also good for balancing gut bacteria.

However, consider what I say about milk and its calcium value on page 141. Bear in mind that a glass of good quality freshly juiced carrot, has the same quantity of calcium as a glass of milk, only the carrot juice assimilates with the body and the milk doesn't.

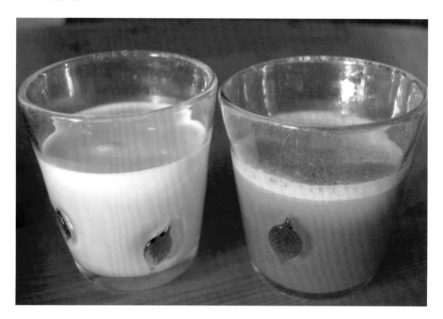

<u>REMEMBER</u>
Milk and carrot juice contain similar amounts of calcium

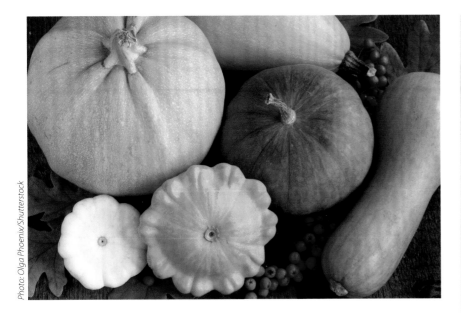

Photo: Olga Phoenix/Shutterstock

Apple cider vinegar
Apple cider vinegar's properties are vast and vary from fighting infection to brightening our teeth. It is theorized to assist weight loss by stabilising blood sugar levels and it can even alleviate post exercise fatigue. Opt for a cloudy, organic, raw version and mix a spoonful into juices or soups or try diluted with water before a meal to help repress the appetite.

Why balsamic vinegar?
Balsamic vinegar unlike other vinegars, doesn't come from fermented grape but from the juice of the grape called the 'must'. It is the process of boiling the must that makes the syrupy texture which is then left in wooden barrels to mature. Choose your vinegars well to ensure it is pure and without additions.

Also, if you want to fill up more because you feel a bit shaky, add in the butternut squash and other pumpkin varieties. If slimming down is more your aim for now, try to hold back from the pumpkin family just a little longer.

Different food types take different times to digest. It makes sense that where possible we think about the order in which we eat food. For instance fruit digests quite quickly, taking about 30 minutes. Meat takes much longer, about 2 or more hours.

If you were to eat fruit salad after a meat dish or most other food choices, you may feel bloated while the fruit just sits in a traffic jam behind the previous course. This also means absorption of nutrients isn't as efficient.

Ideally, for comfort and relieving the digestion, aim to eat in this order:

- fruit
- carbohydrates, (starchy vegetables and all grains, to be introduced later)
- proteins

New food to introduce *(list 2 page 48):*

- spices and herbs
- all variations of pulses
- balsamic vinegar and apple cider vinegar (see side panels)
- soft fruits: blueberries, strawberries, raspberries and peaches
- live organic cow, sheep or goat's yoghurt
- pineapple
- all legumes, white and red kidney beans
- also think of using fennel, watercress, dandelion and parsley too

Day 5

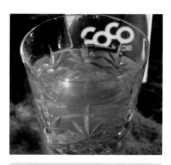

What are electrolytes?

Electrolyte is a term used for salts, specifically ions. The body's fluids such as blood, plasma and the fluid between the cells is a balance made up of these salts: sodium, potassium, chloride, calcium, magnesium, bicarbonate, phosphate and sulphate. For normal cell and organ function, a good balance of electrolytes is essential and this is a key factor to this plan. Imbalance causes disruptions in health from as mild as bloating to critical issues.

Workout day today! This should be your third session so your mind and muscles will have started to get used to the moves.

Be strict with your rest time between exercises, it should be minimal. Make sure all that you need is set up for an uninterrupted few minutes of body blasting!

Have you ever drunk coconut water? It is excellent for many reasons. It is the closest thing in the natural plant world to resemble our blood plasma. It is an excellent re-hydration drink as it is loaded with electrolytes, which is what the body's natural mineral balance requires. It therefore makes an excellent after-exercise drink and one you'd benefit from introducing into your diet now.

Another of coconut water's great qualities is that it is a natural antidote for parasites and bad gut bacteria. While we are cleaning up our eating habits, take it a stage further and get rid of any unwanted guests residing *chez vous*. Parasites are insidious and cause irksome health problems that are hard to pinpoint. They love a rotten soil, an unhealthy diet and are very fond of sugar. Let's starve them and clear them away and leave the more helpful bacteria to work alone.

However, these properties of coconut water are true only of young green coconuts. You'll be lucky to find a young green coconut in less than tropical places but you can buy the coconut water from good health shops and some supermarkets. Just make sure it is pure and without any additions. This will also save you from drilling out a hole in a real coconut – leave that to the indigenous people! They will have a technique that won't be as messy as ours!

Other foods that help with moving on bad bacteria are:

- grapefruits
- ginger
- garlic
- onions
- coconut oil

Eating such foods will give your system a better chance when you are exposed to different environments and climates. So get chopping onions and garlic and add them raw to your meals.

The yoghurt and balsamic were probably a welcome introduction yesterday. These two additions can really spruce up dishes. Go easy on the yoghurt and make absolutely sure it is a 'live' organic yoghurt with 'cultures'.

If you started this plan on a Monday, prepare well for the weekend, be well stocked up and treat it like every other day this week.

Get some more days behind you of this clean eating and you will be well armed against temptations. You are through the hardest part, just keep your seatbelts tightened a little longer!

Day 6

How are you? Looking clearer, feeling giddy but still on track? Well done!

The body is working well getting back into a healthy equilibrium. You may still feel a little short on energy if you're an active type but be patient, your energy will return … two fold! Your body is still getting used to the new 'fuel' and is just dealing with more pressing issues, like purging and healing!

See this like you've gone GREEN!

These past days have been such a good rest for your insides, especially the liver. Think of that throughout this plan. A slight slip up in food choices will be clocked by your liver. It is the detox house of the body and works extremely hard daily, year in year out. Now it is having a rest, well at least working less frantically. See it like an animal in hibernation, don't trouble it and let it restore itself slowly.

Keep to the plan! We're trying for 100% here. Then we will move on to more realistic and sustainable habits. So keep giving it your best, the worst hurdle is over.

Take a look at your eating journal. Would your liver approve of what you've been eating so far?

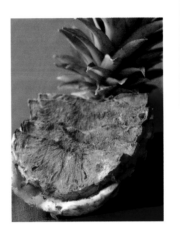

You won't want to undo your good work so keep to the plan and tips to make this as easy as possible for yourself, even if it is the weekend. Keeping on track during these first four weeks is essential to changing habits long-term.

PERSONAL POINT

When I was in the height of competing and racing, I'd have a killer appetite for starch. The training was intensive at three to four sessions per day and my next best interest was eating. I'd knock down a six-pack of hot cross buns, without shame. I also had a penchant for sweet things. I knew I was deluded, but I convinced myself I'd 'burn' it all off in training.

It wasn't until a lady that I greatly respected in the fitness world enlightened me to how sugar (including starchy food) would be destroying my muscle. It was so simply put and it made me think. I'd scoffed my whole life, trained like a Trojan and

for my efforts in the latter, deserved to look like a goddess but I didn't. All this energy expended in trying to build strength, and muscle was wasted by my eating habits. It was also causing stress to my system, not to mention creating extra blubber that according to my exercise regime, shouldn't have been there. I'd been sabotaging myself and having to put in more hours of training to make up for that.

This was the turning point for me. I really understood how, with correct eating, a healthy, toned, fit body can be achieved in minutes rather than hours of hard slog.

Day 7

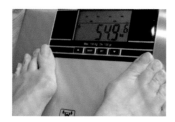

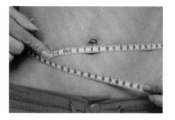

You've been going a week now and you may well be talking of weight loss, looser waistbands and feeling brighter. And you've got more good things to come.

If fat loss was one of your goals and you've shed the extra kilos already, please still keep strictly to the plan. There are plenty more benefits to come and the body needs more time to expose these. I'll tell you about cell renewal a little later on, it will motivate you to keep this up.

If the weekend had the odd hiccup … let it be. Don't be hard on yourself. Just use the next snack or meal as an opportunity to get back on track. Don't start skipping meals or snacks in an effort to balance the errors out. It doesn't work like that. Remember we have to keep fuelling the fire to keep it burning and to keep insulin levels steady.

Take a look at your goals you wrote down at the beginning. Do you feel you're a few steps closer to them now? You may want to refresh them. Write down more, if you are ready to expand on the initial goals. Picture them vividly, see them in colour and motion, write them down on the Personal Notes page at the back of the book or keep them in your day bag for a reminder and reviver.

General condition

Some of you may still be feeling the effects of having a clear out. Among other things, for some they say their skin erupts a little. This is all good … the toxins have to make their way out somehow. When we overload the system with our bad habits the body is constantly trying to rebalance and correct, this is very draining on our immune system. When we give it more of a break, as we are now, it gets more of an opportunity to purge rather than fight urgent matters!

How about that eating journal? Keep writing down everything that goes into your mouth!

And the workout? Are you happy with the level you've been following? Or maybe you need to upgrade a level? Towards the middle and end of the workout you should be quite breathless and unable to string a sentence together in one breath. Are you working hard enough? If not, make sure that you are executing each exercise perfectly. Speed isn't necessarily best with exercise, but performance is! However, don't hang about between each different exercise. Instead, move on to the following exercise swiftly. This will maximise the effect of the plan.

Day 8

Hopefully by now you are fitting into the routine of your new eating habits and feeling brighter. Maybe you are even fitting into clothes you haven't for a little while?

As I've said before, make sure you are eating enough. Don't wait for hunger. That is probably a sign that the body will start slowing down to accommodate the lack of nourishment.

Breakfasts may be feeling a bit thin and you may have had enough of omelettes, eggs and eggs! Remember that too much of anything isn't good. Perhaps include some fish. Look for fish that has nothing added to it other than salt.

Try a smoothie

Throw your choice of fruit in, squeeze an orange, put a dollop of yoghurt, a sprinkle of nuts and blend. Adding fluids to your food gives the feeling of fullness for longer. This isn't the same as drinking with your meal but actually water blended with the food.

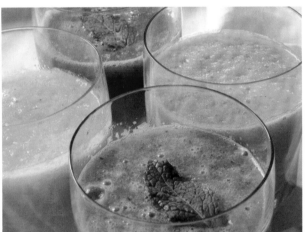

Fruit and vegetable smoothies

That is why soups feel satisfying, as water blended with solid food swells in the digestion. When it is blended, it can't pass through the system quickly. The same plate of food but blended with water reduces signals of hunger. However, I'm not encouraging you to eat less and find tricks to feel full. I'd rather you ate often and enough.

For the protein balance, try adding hemp (more about hemp tomorrow) or ground almonds to the smoothies, or choose something else from the protein list. I know there is discussion over the quality of organic food. But since we are detoxing for this duration, avoid all pesticides and poor quality animal meat where possible.

Even though you've got the hang of this, for now, keep the eating journal up to date. It as important to your success early on, as later in the plan. It is extremely noticeable how those who've kept the journal going keep good momentum throughout.

You're doing so well. And if you're getting compliments on looking good, believe them!

Day 9

You've seen it on the food list and by now you'll know it is a protein. But what is so special about hemp?

It is an easily digested protein and some of its qualities are a great source for mopping up free radical scavengers. It is packed with essential fatty acids (of a perfect ratio) and contains minerals that we can't find easily in other foods; magnesium for one.

Other wonderful things hemp helps with

- detoxification
- speeding up recovery
- improving brain power
- digesting other nutrients
- promoting healthy gut bacteria
- balancing hormones

What's a free radical?

Free radicals are destructive entities that, over time, lead to ageing.

Simply put, the body is made up of atoms or nuclei of atoms. Surrounding these nuclei of atoms are electrons, which work in pairs. Occasionally a pair of electrons separate leaving the atom without a pair.

The atom is then very reactive and known as a free radical.

When cells in the body frequently encounter free radicals they become damaged, aged and eventually the organism dies.

And because it helps to balance hormones, it can therefore help with getting the body to naturally reach its perfect weight. It also contains Vitamins E and A, calcium, iron and zinc. It really is a super food squared! The only thing less than super about it is that the supermarkets don't stock it. You'll need to get it from a healthfood shop or order some online. Either way, buy some! Go for the shelled hemp seed as it is easier to mix into salads, grains and juices. Keep it well sealed and use it generously.

It would be easy to overload on animal protein during these weeks if you weren't paying attention to filling up enough with vegetables. Too much animal protein can be draining on the body and in extremes, our health. BUT that doesn't mean we shouldn't eat it. Protein is essential, but selection is important. Make sure you are varying your protein choices.

Make sure you get a workout in today. Give it your all and then ask yourself if you're ready to move up a level to something more intensive.

Your body will really be starting to respond to all the exercise now. Even if you don't see the benefit yet, it will be quietly working its changes.

Day 10

Day 10 and see how well you are doing!

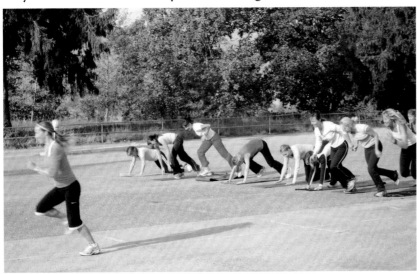

If you were with me doing the courses that I run, I just know the changes in you would now be obvious to an outsider; clearer eyes and skin, tighter body shape and generally more vitality.

So much has been going on within you lately that it can't help but show on the outside now. But there is plenty more of this to come so keep going, keep to the plan, keep letting your body optimise itself all it can.

Now would be a good time to get out your list of goals that you added to a few days ago. Part of achieving a goal is to take action every day … every day. For us that is healthy eating, exercising and whatever else that was relevant on your list.

Think of that statistic … you are 100 times more likely to achieve your goal if you write it down. Get three more goals down on paper today. Anything that feels right for you, whether that be a short-term or long-term project, write them down nice and clear. As emphasised in the 'Getting Started' chapter, use the present tense, as if today you already have what you are aiming for.

Is your diet varied enough?

Keep trying new choices on the lists even if they wouldn't normally be your first choice. It is important to vary the nutritional sources and who knows, by now you may enjoy the taste more.

Take time at some point each day to plan your meals. Our recipes are mostly quick and simple and will satisfy your need for interesting tastes.

A couple of moments of thought and planning makes this all the more achievable and enjoyable.

My goals
* I am getting to bed earlier
* My stomach doesn't feel bloated
* I am enjoying the extra exercise

Day 11

You'll be well into the rhythm of things now. Just keep organised, keep on top of snacks and prepare for the day whether you are home or out and about.

Being prepared makes a huge difference to how successful you are and, importantly, keeping the blood sugar levels nice and steady.

If there is a slip up or a 'bad moment', just leave it behind you and get back on track with the next meal or snack. You know what to do: snack with your vegetable or fruit choices and get some protein in too.

Make this easy for yourself, you now know how to.

Food to introduce today *(list 3 page 48)*

- More soft fruits: **apricots, blackberries, blackcurrants, cherries, cranberries, grapes, plums and redcurrants.**
- Get some new texture and taste with **beetroot and radishes.**
- Grains: **oatmeal and oatflakes, buckwheat, barley and millet.**
  The flours of these grains will come in later. For now keep these to the minimum and try them on alternate days.
- **Rice, oat, spelt and almond milk in moderation.** These will add interest to the above grains. Vanilla flavoured rice milk can have a pleasant taste but check the ingredients are free of sugar or syrups. Use these where you used to use cow's/goat's/sheep's milk.
- **Soy sauce:** make sure you use all natural ingredients.
- **Smoked fish e.g. salmon and mackerel.**
- **Crunchy flaked soya:** use in moderation for texture.

REMEMBER

Don't skip meals or snacks to make up for a less than great food choice. That will just make it harder for you.

Often, after some types of food, we're still left feeling hungry and with the taste for something else, so watch out for that.

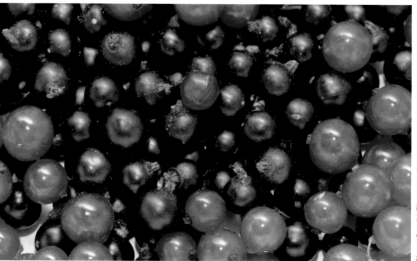

Photo: Serg64/Shutterstock

Go easy on the portions. Start with just a couple of spoonfuls of grains. It is very important to gradually reintroduce new food. Also try one day with grains, the next day without (see page 147).

Today is an exercise day. How are you managing to fit it into your day? How about you getting up and on with it before anything else, even breakfast? This is such a good time to workout, especially now that you'll be waking up feeling fresher than you used to.

More information **Benefits of the 'First Thing Workout'**

- The stomach is empty and so there is no need to wait and postpone a workout until a meal has digested
- It sparks up energy levels well for the day
- It sparks up the metabolism for the day
- More body fat is used for energy
- There's no need to try to fit the workout in later on
- And … you can jump into easy wear kit, do the workout and shower after!
- Whatever your chosen exercise time, commit to it as if it is a meeting that you must attend!

You are close to half way now and look at the good results you've already created! You can look forward to more of these.

Keep going!

Day 12

I'm sure you'll be noticing improvements since you've thrown yourself into this.

Hopefully you'll be feeling proud of how far you've come as far as change of habits and a few evident results. If you've got this far by keeping to the plan, pat yourself on the back as no doubt there have been temptations before you.

You should know that you are also well on your way. You wouldn't want to go back on any of that discipline and clearing out now, would you?

Everybody's fat loss is different

Therefore timing of fat loss can vary from person to person. Much as we can bank on good results, we can't bank on the timing of them. Mostly people lose weight in the first week of this plan but if this isn't you, don't fret. Sometimes for others, during the second week the speed of fat loss may seem to have slowed. Again stay confident, the body is still working away to create a healthy balance so, evident or not, good things are happening. Ultimately we're interested in the end result, not the different stages.

If you were not used to eating regularly before this plan, it can be that the metabolism is getting used to its new responsibilities. In some cases, eating more speeds up the metabolism, but the adjustment to speeding up may take a while and there will probably be a period when you'll be concerned that you could be over eating! Have faith that the metabolism does find its optimum efficiency. It just needs to trust you will feed it regularly with nutritious, calming food.

So, if you used to eat erratically, the idea that eating regularly will eventually slim you down, may be a difficult concept to accept. You may well be consuming more calories than usual but all these calories are from food that the body can assimilate and digest. I've been podgier living off 1,000 calories per day from a bowl of rice krispies and chocolate bars than 2,500 calories of real food. Let's face it, you can eat too much pizza, bread and cakes but can you eat too many vegetables?

Your eating journal will be an honest reference for you. Looking back, you'll understand how you found your way to feeling and looking so good.

Stick with what we're doing here. It is worth it.

You may well find that you hit a plateau at 2 weeks – that happens! That's when you have to stay focused on your goals and maintain your motivation! Remember this is so short in the grand scheme of things so let's stick to it as well as we can.

Weight loss is like this: you will lose different amounts every week and you will stay the same some weeks.

Day 13

Hopefully you are starting to feel great now. You may not even recognise it but take yourself back a few weeks. How were your levels of energy throughout the day? And your moods? And what about sleeping, is that better?

Things should be much more stable now, even if the world around you is rattling!

Some people lose a few kilos by now and some, like me, are slower. I usually lose a kilo in the first week but what I'm more interested in is the change of condition. Fitness levels and muscle condition are vastly improved even in this short time. That is because the body has been fuelled with a diet of clean foods rather than the odd chocolate Florentine or two … now there is nothing impairing its day-to-day functions so it can operate so much better. What you are doing makes a difference in how the skin or flesh sits too. Extra bits won't hang like they used to and everything will tighten up a tweak.

What is so bad about caffeine?

You know that kick or rush you get after a cuppa? This is adrenaline. You may have got so immune to it in the past that you no longer felt that buzz. Regardless of feeling it or not, coffee makes the body release adrenaline. Adrenaline gives a boost or a high but it is nothing more than a prelude to a slump or low. You've probably heard of the 'fight or flight' expression. This is used to describe the release of adrenaline that comes to man or creature in a fearful situation. It is a surge of energy instantly provided to cope with a crisis, meaning the individual can fight his way out or flee.

However drinking a cup of caffeine isn't usually a terrifying experience so there is no need to flee. But the chemical change still comes about. This change triggers the production of insulin, the very thing that provides the energy to get up and go. But mostly we don't run for our lives after a dose of caffeine, we get on with normal duties with a bit of a lift or a buzz. Yet once the insulin is released into the bloodstream, it can't return from where it came. So what can it do, where can it go? It encourages the body to lay down this surplus energy as FAT, also inhibiting the break down of fat.

The rapid changes in blood sugar levels after this experience of caffeine leaves the caffeine drinker seeking another kick and brings on hunger. So it is unlikely in this state that the coffee drinker will reach out for healthy foods! Coffee and any caffeine ingredient is a stimulant. Start to see it as that. Eating regularly as you are, with the combination of foods listed, will curb the desire for stimulants.

Keep to the plan, we'll be adding more changes shortly but stick to this for now.

Have you planned your exercise time for today?

REMEMBER

Keep remembering we're giving our systems a rest from working overtime from more challenging foods. We're combining that with instigating slow but sure fat loss – hence the low complex carbs and protein ratio.

A healthy approach to food is key. Those who eat for health get slim. Those who eat to be slim, struggle.

Remove the 'fattening' and 'slimming' food thinking and swap it for nourishing or not!

Green tea

Green tea also contains caffeine. Yet the production of the leaf is different from that of other tea leaves; the caffeine content doesn't raise the blood pressure like other sources of caffeine do.

Green tea has many qualities so if it is to your liking, keep drinking it.

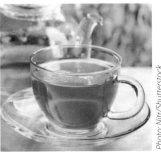

Photo: Nitr/Shutterstock

Day 14

If you started this plan early in the week, how was the weekend? Were you faced with any temptations or were they easier to resist than normal?

Remember this isn't an 'on a diet' and then 'come off a diet' plan. We're just giving the body the best chance to clean up, respond well and do what it is meant to do.

Weigh and measure yourself today and log it in your Notes and Progress pages.

Even if you've hit your desired weight, keep going. There will have been weight loss in these early stages but you're yet to enjoy the change in condition. See how much improvement there has been in this short time, square it, and you'll be positively glowing in a couple more weeks.

Have a think about this to keep your motivation up:

- 98% of the atoms in your body have changed in the past year
- every 3 months your bones are renewed – well the atoms passing through the cells have renewed
- the skin only takes a month to renew
- the stomach lining is constantly changing and after 4 days it has a new one
- the liver's cells turn very slowly but as you've already heard, after 6 weeks it can be regenerated

See this as an opportunity to optimise your insides and outside! Keep up with the body's fast turn over, keep fuelling it well. With that speed of regeneration and this much green living, we'll be good as new at a very deep level!

To really boost results, get exercising everyday now. There is a quick workout option in the exercise section designed as a filler. It only takes a moment, will barely get you into a sweat but will ensure that your body is burning fuel well and effectively, i.e. burning fat. Do your utmost to alternate the regular workouts with the filler workout from now on.

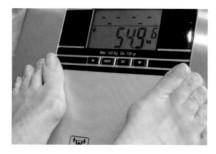 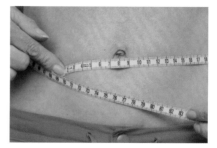

Keep going!

Day 15

You are more than halfway now and there are plenty more positive results to come. See what you have achieved in such a short time! Imagine how much more you can achieve in the next half of this plan.

Any lurking ailments could be well behind you now. Just think back … did you struggle coming round in the morning? Felt a little groggy? Did you have any irritations that you just put up with like coughs, sniffles, aches, ulcers or other persistent symptoms?

Assessing your goals and determining your thoughts

Now have another think about your goals. Visualise exactly how you want to feel and look by the time this plan is over. How much energy will you have? How will you fit into clothes?

Take it an image further. Can you hear compliments from others too? See it, feel it, hear it … get these thoughts on to paper now. Our thoughts determine so much, so make these thoughts come alive.

Give them an airing outside your own head! Write them down. They may not be fitness or flat tummy related but, while you're in this great frame of mind of self-control and discipline, work it to the end. Put them on paper, think them through and take action … daily.

This plan has inspired so many people to hold the reins tighter on their health and fitness and get what they can out of themselves. Ride on this wave of positivity!

My thoughts
* *Feeling brighter. Looking brighter and fresher*
* *My body all tidied up in shape, condition and health*
* *Steady energy and hormones … calm and sweet dreams*

Get the right exercise

Are you doing the right exercise level for yourself? If you started on the first level, you'll be ready to go to intermediate level now.

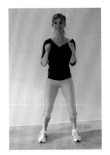 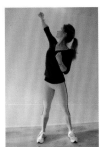 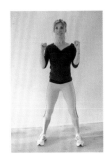 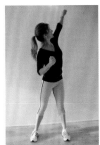

Keep pushing yourself. These are short exercise sessions and are meant to be quite intense, make sure you get the most out of this plan!

Day 16

At this point the first phase of the plan should certainly be taking effect:

- The nutrition value of your food choices has increased
- Your organs and insides will be reaping the rewards of your efforts
- The metabolism will be working well as you've kick-started mobilising surplus fat

Compared to lots of things in the world of now, nature changes slowly and your body is a piece of nature. But it is doing a thorough job, from the inside out. It's important to appreciate that even though there will be periods when it seems like nothing is happening, beneath your skin there is a lot of correcting and healing occurring.

Remember, results take time. Nonetheless by now:

- you'll have more energy
- muscle tone is improving
- the metabolism is increasing

A food tip

Bean sprouts or mung beans as you may know them, are packed with energy and goodness. They contain vitamin A, C and even have a small amount of protein. They are also high in a valuable component, B17.

What does B17 do? It rebalances cells to a healthy state. In fact some claim it selectively destroys cancer cells. Look out for this magic food (even better, grow the sprouts yourself) and mix it into salads and vegetable servings. Eat them raw.

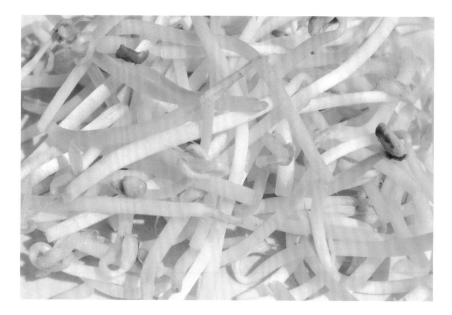

REMEMBER

One month of clean living can clear up one year of damage. Be dedicated to this objective.

Day 17

Hopefully you are feeling proud. You should be. Maybe it hasn't been without the occasional stumble but I hope you would agree, it is a huge upgrade in self-care nonetheless.

It is important that you have enough variety of nutrients. We can get a bit stuck on certain dishes and habits … same fruit, same vegetables and meat. Keep an eye on that. Your eating habits are much cleaner than before so optimise this period of easy absorption, with variety … .from the list of course! More food will come in soon.

Look at your protein options

- Have you had liver lately?
- Or a food rich in iron, lots of parsley or shell fish?
- Vary your salads: some leaves offer more than others, but in short, keep rotating your food and nutrients

Acid vs alkaline

There is some information for you about acid and alkaline balance on page 90. Now that you have adopted these healthier habits, it would be a good time to consider which foods are alkaline and which are acidic. It isn't always obvious. Some foods seem acidic but in digestion become alkaline. For instance, lemon is alkaline in digestion and oats tip towards acidic. More on that later.

Remember that 50% of energy goes into digestion, the other 50% goes into renewal. So keep the task easy for your body. Exercise, rest, mental composure, attitude to life and food, all have a balance in this.

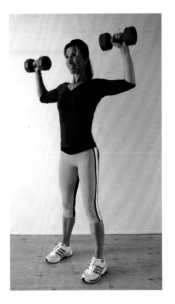

REMEMBER

If you have kept to the plan, today will be an exercise day with your weights or other resistance equipment.

Work each muscle with control and imagine every muscle fibre working. Put some mind into that body!

More information **Digestion**

Many people who followed this plan found that excretion and faeces changed at some stage.

Naturally, with a change of eating habits the faeces do change but for some it was more particular and most noticeable after a couple of weeks or more into the tidy up.

There may be a stronger odour and a film of mucus. This would suggest that the bowels are really clearing out any old debris that hasn't passed the large intestines thoroughly. Mucus builds up on the intestinal tract wall over years, even with a half healthy diet. This stagnant stuff is internal pollution and a breeding ground for unfavourable bacteria. It is best flushed out and away, be grateful it is gone! Read more about this in the 'Queries and Questions' section (page 142).

Day 18

My goals

* *I am sleeping well + my body is regenerating + rejuvenating*

**I am slimmer with toned muscles and fresher, younger skin*

**I have much more vitality, energy and mental clarity*

Meeting with myself
Organisation and preparation
Where am I now? Behind.
What do I need to do to improve on this? Buy healthy food and sort out snacks for the day.
What are the steps that I need to take? Pack snacks after dog walk – think ahead.
What does the end result look like? Pleased, in order and on top of things and accepting of interruption.

Discipline and Focus
Where am I now? Average.
Set my goals and clarify aims.
Set times for exercise and stick to healthy eating.
Healthy, good energy levels and mood, all in order.
Health and fitness
Average and behind.
Follow the plan, get on with better habits.
Exercise 5 X per week for 15 minutes, eat food with vitality.
Awake, alive! Sleeping well, good skin, feeling positive with lifted bum!

General balance
Ok, nearly.
Less fun food, be more productive, have more fun.
Book outings with friends and timetable admin work.
Projects finished, good social life, lots of outdoors and nature, healthy body and bank account

18 days of clean eating and we need to keep it that way for a little while yet.

Apart from giving the body its month long rest and recovery time, there is another very important side to keeping on track – changing habits.

It is hard to believe that years of habit forming can actually come to an end. But give the blood sugar levels a chance, give the organs a rest, fuel yourself with goodness that gets the body into fine equilibrium and you'll be impressed with yourself. After these 28 days, the next time your favourite treat is presented to you, it won't have the allure it used to.

Just to make sure you really reach this point and can feel it for yourself, here is a checklist to go through:

1. Is protein at least 10% and at most 30% of each of your meals and snacks?
2. Do you keep your eating journal diary updated?
3. Are you eating regularly, five times a day?
4. With, at the most, three hours between?
5. Are you keeping well-hydrated and sipping lightly throughout the day? See page 139 for hydration.
6. Are you doing the exercises daily now?
7. If not daily, are you exercising at least every other day?
8. Are your meals varied and do they feature foods to assist good gut flora? (see Day 5)
9. Are you focused on your goals and have you got them written down clearly?
10. If you can say 'yes' to all of these, you are doing very well and there is no doubt that you're on your way to a fine figure inside and out.

If not, do you need another 'Meeting with Myself' to ensure complete success?

Exercise today will be the 'filler' workout. Find a few spare minutes and just knock this session out and take another step towards success.

Day 19

How is your motivation? Sometimes we don't think we're doing so well and can focus only on the slip ups rather than the successes. So ask yourself, what have I done today to move closer to my goals?

Keep yourself positive, remind yourself of your achievement so far and the improvements you have made. When you aim high it is easy to forget how far you have already come. There is more good to come so see this through and keep to plan.

Protect your good work! Others may not completely understand your mission or discipline but just remind them it is only for a short duration while you get back on keel. A fellow fitness professional reminded me of a Bill Cosby quote, *"I don't know the key to success, but the key to failure is trying to please everybody"*. So keep to your game plan, not theirs.

Today's exercise will be the resistance workout. Put on some music that makes you want to move and give it your best shot. You may be wondering how such short workouts can make a difference when even the government's exercise recommendation suggest 30 minutes a few times a week. This is a general guide and while any exercise is beneficial over none, it is somewhat outdated.

Endless studies show that long aerobic exercise actually releases the hormone, cortisol (more about this in tomorrow's message), which is counterproductive to fat loss!

Short, sharp, explosive workouts are the way forward for improving your fitness and figure … So make sure that's what your session today feels like!

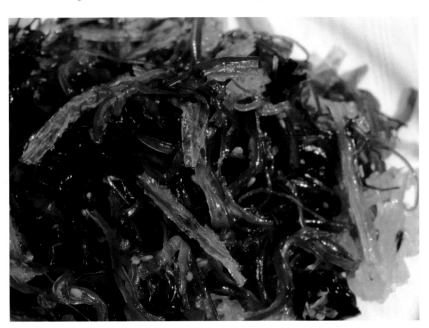

Spruce up your salads with seaweed

There are a few types of algae and between them they offer a variety of nutrients in minerals, vitamins, protein and calcium. It is believed to also be a hormone stabiliser and contain anti-cancerous properties.

Look out for:

Arame – black

Dulse – purply red

Nori – purple or red

Wakame – green

Algae in its real form, is far superior to any manmade dietary supplement that can have an inappropriate balance of extracts, including heavy metals.

Day 20

Poisonous stress

This is how poisonous stress is: in Mike Nash's research he writes of an experiment performed with a man's saliva while he was enraged.

When they analysed the saliva they found it to have the same qualities of a snake's venom. The researchers continued experimenting with this saliva and injected it into a group of small animals. Each one of them died.

It is no coincidence that we find anger and stress so uncomfortable to be close to!

Could stress be affecting my efforts?

Naturally life has its ways of washing up unwanted problems before our eyes and we can feel our stress levels changing. All these outside issues can of course affect how we handle day-to-day jobs, and even sabotage fat loss. You've probably heard the phrase 'stress makes you fat'. But you may have witnessed something else, that stress has made you lose weight! There may well have been weight loss, but as pointed out in the earlier part of this plan, what kind of weight loss was that? Most likely muscle and quite likely there was fat gain around your midsection.

Unfortunately we can't mask our stresses from the body and in states of stress the adrenal glands release cortisol which in turn increases insulin levels. (See page 134 to be reminded of insulin's effect on health). The physical reactions to this are an increased appetite and a slower metabolism. The appetite increases because cortisol effectively numbs you to the hormone leptin, which is the very hormone that tells you when you've eaten enough. This is why a good protein is essential in healthy eating, as it encourages the release of leptin.

So back to the stress part. Stress can set off this chemical reaction that sets you up for eating things that, in turn, make you more stressed and hold fat!

Cortisol also eats away at your vital tissue, muscle. As you know, muscle among other things, is valuable in terms of improved circulation and keeping our fat percentages low. The more muscle we have, the more calories we burn, the less fat we have. It also weighs three times more than fat. So think back to if you were ever stressed and skinny. Were you muscle and bones or fat and bones? After sickness, crash diets or rapid weight loss, the weight comes back on quickly due to the muscles regaining their volume. Whereas with true fat loss the weight doesn't come back because fat is slow to lay down … just as it is slow to shift. So we create our own cortisol whether it be through habits or stress. The important thing now is to keep stress levels down. Easier said than done. But the other option is much less favourable!

- Keep a good alkaline balance in your food (see Day 21 for more on this).
- Get enough magnesium. Hemp is rich in this. Also dark greens, seafood, almonds, and oily seeds and nuts are other sources.
- Get a few minutes of sun or natural light every day.
- Try calming herbs and teas. Camomile, peppermint and liquorice are good for easing digestion.
- Relax! It is the most obvious one and the most essential. Insist on a few minutes every day doing something that transports your mind elsewhere: reading, gardening, meditating, a relaxing bath, whatever works for you.
- Get things into perspective. Most stresses aren't life or death but mere aggravations that we allow to pollute our health and humour!

Day 21

Just a few more days of our clean out remain and here are a few new tastes to add in. There are more significant additions to come in a few days which will expand your cuisine.

You will see that coconut milk is also on list 4 (page 49). This will really make dishes more interesting. Coconut milk is rather misunderstood and you may have heard that it has high cholesterol content. However, after consuming coconut milk, the body's cholesterol level is not elevated. It would appear that the body recognises the coconut's composition as friendly.

Although this is a month-long programme, I hope you will be adopting some of these habits for the long-term. You will notice further changes over the months if you maintain certain points that we have highlighted in these pages and over your current programme. Something to take a look at now is the balance of acidic and alkaline foods, and how these affect us.

As we have noticed, limiting the heavier carbs (rice, pasta, pastries) from our diet brings more consist energy. Try all you can to keep the vegetable and salad quantities high, even when you re-introduce some of these carbs.

Acidic foods

Acidic forming foods can cause and aggravate inflammatory conditions in the body. These may come through as skin, joint, bladder or digestive problems. The body does try to excrete residues of acid forming foods through perspiration, urine and breath, but obviously any overload means the body slows down to accommodate and deal with the accumulation.

Getting the balance right, or at least being mindful of improving it, can assist greatly in many health matters, not least fat loss. As you know by now, cells bloat when the chemical balance is wrong. Anything that stalls the body's normal workload will compromise aspects such as vitality while perpetuating fat storage.

The taste of the food won't tell you if it is alkaline or acidic. For instance lemons seem acidic but are alkaline to the body. Meats are alkaline until digested when they become acidic. Overcooked food is more acidic. As ever, raw vegetables assimilate better than cooked ones. Vegetable juices will greatly help with the alkaline balance. There is more about raw product and juices in the days ahead.

Water can help neutralise the balance, and a squeeze of lemon or lime in the water will too.

Weigh and measure yourself today and note it down with the other records.

If today is part of a slow week in terms of fat loss or other progress, be reminded of the body's intelligence and its constant regeneration, visible or not.

New additions

Consider: fresh figs, coconut and, if you rather buy stock than make it, look for an all natural ingredients one.

If figs are in season and you enjoy them, get some! Choose fresh and organic where possible. They will spruce up a dish nicely too. Figs are quite rich in minerals, they contain calcium, phosphorous and potassium.

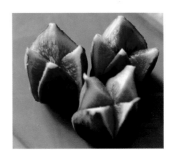

REMEMBER

What can seem a healthy day's intake can be misleading, e.g. porridge for breakfast (oats are acidic), fish, rice and salad for lunch (rice, fish and meat are acidic) etc.

Take a look at page 90 for a rough guide to alkaline and acidic food. There should be no need to make huge dietary changes. Just become aware of your intake and balance and add in food that is more alkaline.

Day 22

Try to have a RAW day this week. 100%.

That will mean a lot of fruit, vegetables, nuts, seeds, hemp and whatever you find works for you from the protein list. Make sure you are stocked up on ginger, garlic and other hot herbs and roots that fight parasites.

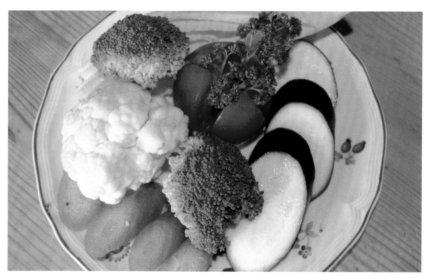

Raw food is rich in enzymes and nutrients.

When we cook food, we boil and bake out a big percentage of their nutrient value. In fact it is more severe than that. To help the intestines digest cooked foods, the body's white blood cells abandon other parts of the body to assist the digestion process.

After years of this, the immune system tires and leaves the rest of the body vulnerable to disease. Most food we buy or prepare is cooked, but that isn't to say it is best. We become very accustomed to soft, cooked foods, yet raw foods make for complete and effective absorption of nutrients.

'Dead food'

Many naturopaths call cooked food 'dead food'. They believe there is no vitality in cooked food and so therefore none is transferred to us. It would be impractical for many to adopt 100% raw eating habits. But, considering a percentage of raw food for each meal would make a marked difference to our health and vitality. Another easy and excellent way to supplement your raw intake is by juicing (more on this on Day 25).

Raw meats and fish may carry unwelcome bacteria. As mentioned above, adding raw garlic, ginger, onions and other naturally hot plants, will make an unfriendly environment for these parasites. Remember parasites and bacteria are within all of us. It is just a matter of having a good flora balance and not to create an environment that parasites will thrive on.

PERSONAL POINT

After my dog got knocked down by a car many years ago, she developed a thyroid problem. The impact had been on her head and affected thyroid function. I was guided towards endless prescriptions, all of which upset her health and happiness.

Instead, I researched what dogs should really eat for optimum health. The findings were obvious really; their meat should be raw, as if just been caught, with grains and vegetables as if found in the digestive tract of their prey. The transformation in her was remarkable; she became a happy, healthy, shiny, fit, fast and well-rested dog. And, against all expert speculation, her thyroid problem rebalanced. If an owner is meant to look like their dog, I'm happy with my look-a-like!

Thanks to raw garlic in every evening meal, there has not been a flea, worm or parasite in 6 years! Noticeably, when the diet slips or she has been drawn to raid the local bins, her coat loses the shine and she can become hormonal and obstinate.

This just goes to show how poor quality or 'dead' food inhibits the absorption of the finer food and nutrients. Don't worry, my health findings aren't based on my dog's health! But with such apparent and obvious visual changes, it helps illustrate the impact that raw and basic food has on reversing sickness and creating a base for vitality.

So pick your raw day, plan your food and make raw food a greater feature.

The last week now, pull out all the stops!

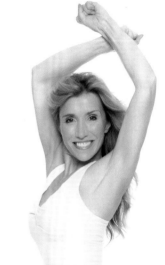

Photo: Andres Lesauvage

Day 23

Why no wheat or bread yet?

Wheat can create problems for some stomachs. You may know of someone who is wheat sensitive or reacts badly to it. Actually the news here is that if we, or bakeries, were to use slow-acting yeast there wouldn't be a problem.

The slow-acting yeast would work away at the dough and aid the digestion of wheat, making it easy for our consumption and digestion. However most of what we encounter is fast-acting yeast. That means wheat isn't 'treated' as much, if at all, by the active yeast. And therein lies the problem.

So aside from the intolerance problems that some grains can cause, it has been noticeable with my groups if I introduce grains or bread too soon in to the plan, it is harder to pull off 'tidying the temple' to the end, and beyond. There is more success in fat loss, vitality, curbing cravings and discipline beyond the 28 day plan, if we have a longer stint without these foods.

However, on Day 26 there will be more food to introduce. Some of these are flours and grains.

Have you decided on your raw day yet? Once you have tried it out be sure to include a percentage of raw fresh 'plant' food every day.

How about your goals? Any more you'd like to add? Have you ticked off our first few yet? Could you be a dress size smaller?

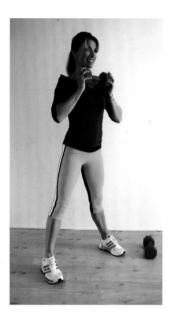

REMEMBER

By this stage your muscles will be familiar with the moves and repetitions.

So make sure each resistance exercise is executed slowly and fully so that you can be sure of using every one of those muscle fibres for fine toning.

PERSONAL POINT

Keep on top of your eating journal.

It is easy to feel very confident by now about what and when you are eating. From experience this can tend to be a stage when, because you know exactly what you are doing, it isn't such a big deal if you slack off here and there. But it is!

By 'slacking off', I mean the contrary of what it implies (treats and cheats) and actually **not eating enough** or **often enough.** If this happens, the body can look a little drawn while the muscles are somewhat empty and deflated, the perky colouring in the skin can go too. A short time like this would also have you steering towards foods and 'pick me ups' that will put out your glow!

So back to the eating journal … note things down. How do your eating habits compare with a couple of weeks ago? Keep those reins tight and see this through, eating correctly and sufficiently.

Day 24

What changes do I notice? This is a question you can regularly ask yourself as it helps to keep a good perspective on how you are really doing. It may be, you feel that today or yesterday wasn't so great in terms of keeping a good handle on the plan. But could it be your standards have changed and your expectations are higher than a few weeks ago? Just remind yourself of how you used to eat and be aware that you are making progress!

It is time to appreciate your success and all the knowledge and application that has come with it.

Take your mind back to any irksome complaints that you had before … tickly coughs, poor sleep patterns, skin conditions etc. Are they behind you now?

It has been the accumulation of improved habits that have made these differences to you. Don't underestimate how even small changes now and into the future will make significant long-term changes.

Thinking ahead for your health and taking steps now will build a good foundation for days, months and years ahead. It is these steps now, in every part of life, that breed fortune or failure. Luck and loss cannot be avoided, as I understand so well, but a sound foundation can be built for your wellbeing, from now onwards.

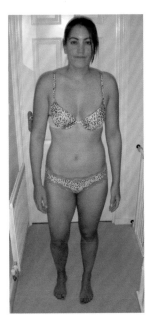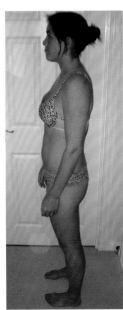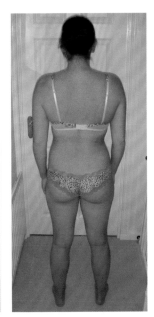

Have a look at your 'before' shot and have a good look in the mirror. How have you changed?

At this stage there will be some encouraging changes and more to come … keep motivated and carry on.

Day 25

If you have a juicer, get it out, dust it off and remind yourself how it works.

Get the most out of juicing

Juicing is the fast track to health and a great way of consuming not just the recommended amount of raw portions but lots of vitamins. As emphasised before, getting live enzymes into the gut is one of the best steps to health.

The easiest way of doing this is through your juicer. If you haven't got one, get one and spend good money on it too. It'll be a false health economy to spend £50 only to find it doesn't extract all the juice, is rather fiddly to wash up and not robust.

Another point to consider is that if you are going to juice handfuls of fruit and veg, you want to make sure you are getting all the goodness. Good juicers, turn slowly and don't generate heat which all works towards conserving the nutrients. If you are able take the plunge and get a heavy-duty industrial one for £250 or more, you won't regret it and it'll serve gallons of juice for years. A good juicer will leave a dry pulp which you can use for thickening soups, gravies or as I do, add to the dog's meal.

The benefits of juicing

One juice could contain more than you'd consume in a few days of raw food. For example, how often do you eat 3 carrots, 2 sticks of celery, 4 large green leaves, half a pepper and a chunk of cabbage, in one sitting? Imagine the boost a couple of juices a day could bring. It is the quickest way to get live enzymes to the stomach and goodness to the blood stream. It is as fast as alcohol in reaching these parts.

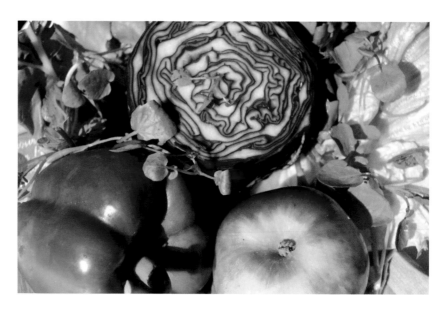

Due to the speed with which they are absorbed, raw juices save energy on the digestive track. As previously mentioned, 50% of our energy goes into digesting foods which is why fasting now and again, especially during sickness, is considered good for health. Since fasting is rather hard for most of us (and not a great deal of fun!) juicing is your next best option. Holistic practitioners have been known to put some patients on 12 juices a day and have incredible stories in turning around serious illnesses.

A few tips

- Drink the juice immediately to acquire all the benefits.
- Also bear in mind that a lot of juiced fruit still equates as sugar to the body.
- Try to keep the fruit low and the vegetables high.
- A small vanity tip – if you're juicing a lot, you may want to drink it through a straw to avoid the teeth discolouring.

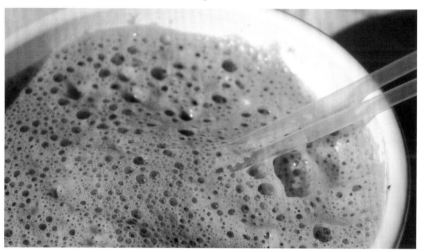

REMEMBER

Nutritious as juicing is, don't rely on the vitamin boost for fibre. Since we are not fasting during this time, we still need the bulk of fresh vegetable produce to aid bowel movement.

A great boosting and liver support juice is a combination of the following:

- ¼ of a small red cabbage (this contains vitamin C and good amount of potassium)
- ½ a green pepper (rich in vitamin A, C and potassium)
- Romaine lettuce (two times more potassium than a loose leaf lettuce and quite high levels of folic acid)
- watercress (rich in vitamin A)
- 1 apple (this makes all the rest more palatable!)

This is a great mix of nutrients, I can't promise a great taste though! But you'll feel quite a bit brighter straight after.

REMEMBER

Even beyond tidying your temple time, think twice in the future about sports drinks off the shelves. They can contain ingredients that may actually deplete the body of minerals and in addition, upset the acid and alkaline balance.

A good après-sports juice to replace lost minerals would be a mix of:

- curly kale, which is high in alkaline quality and helps neutralise lactic acid build up (the burning sensation in muscles)
- cucumber and celery (for sodium)

Day 26

Hopefully snacks have become completely routine to you now. But are they lacking variety?

While nuts and fruit are easy for travel and putting in pockets, there are other options you can pick from. Get yourself a mini Tupperware pot and let this be your saviour from having to stop at garages and searching for the best of some less than healthy options.

To make snacks a little more interesting, you could start bringing in crisp breads or crackers made up from the grain options from the list below. This way you can place a piece of meat or fish with a slice of tomato or salad. More grains can come in later after the 28 days and open up the crisp bread options.

Keep an eye on the crisp bread consumption. It would be easy to squeeze out valuable snacks like raw vegetables in replacement for a cracker. Habits start step by small step and, over time, manifest their impact on our health, both good and bad (read 'Our Little Habits' chapter on page 134). So keep your snacks broad and varied, spread your net wide so as to get a good amount of vegetables, fruits and all the protein options, animal and/or vegetable.

You may not feel like bringing these things back into your larder just yet. If your quest is further fat loss, leave the new additions until after the 28 days or when you feel ready.

More food

- Peanut or a nut butter (check the ingredients are all natural and without hydrogenated fat)
- Rye and pumpernickel bread
- Barley, buckwheat, chestnut, corn, millet, oat, rye and spelt flour
- Grains: rye, spelt, quinoa and brown rice

If you miss bread you can try making your own (see Rye Bread on page 97 of the recipe section). If yeast is in the recipe make sure that it is slow-acting and allow it to work overnight or certainly for a few hours. Make a batch and freeze some. Always choose wholesome flours as suggested from the list above.

Nice as it will be getting your teeth into the texture of bread again, remember how much space it takes up. It is quite filling. Make sure you don't get short of space and end up compromising on freshly grown produce.

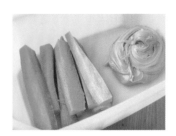

Other things to try

Cucumber, linseeds, mint leaves and yoghurt as an alternative. One of my favourites is raw carrot with a splodge of peanut butter.

Peanut butter? I know I sound like a heathen, but search well in your healthfood shop and you'll find a pure peanut butter, with only oil and salt added.

Day 27

You're one day away form the finish line!

Hopefully you'll want to carry on with much of the way you have been eating these past days but, before we move on from here, remember those self-tests you did at the start of tidying up?

Go back to your notes and see the difference you have made:

1. Lift your shirt up and jiggle in front of the mirror. Does that tummy stop moving when you stop?

2. Pinch your inner thigh. Is it as sensitive as day one?

3. Grab the flesh on the inner thigh. Is it less bumpy, if you had cellulite to start, has it reduced?

4. How is the skin on the backs of the arms and upper outside of the legs? Smoother?

5. Take a look at your skin. Are there shadows beneath your eyes? Are they lighter than before? How is your skin's luminosity?

6. Is your tongue pink and smooth? Is there less of a white covering and fewer cracks?

7. If you had deep, dry cracks on your heels, how are they now?

8. Test your liver, brush the fingers across the right side beneath your ribs. Do the stroke marks fade fast or stay a second or two?

Not all of these points will apply to everyone, but the odd one may. There may have been other ailments that you noted down. How do they compare to now?

Maybe ladies, you have noticed that hormonally, things feel better too. Whether that is menstrual discomfort, PMT or other hormonal upsets.

Assuming you would like to maintain the benefits that you have earned, read the 'Moving on from here' section (page 145).

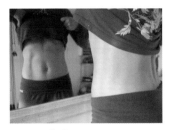

Tummy shake

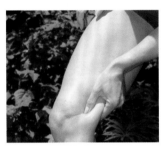

Knee pinch

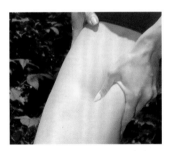

Upper leg

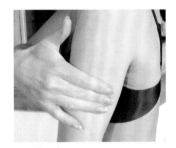

Arm brush

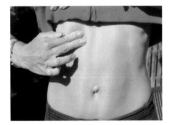

Liver stroke

Day 28

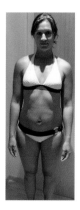
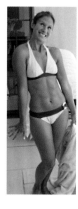

This is the final hurdle and here you are.

Though you will be so in the swing of things it probably won't feel like relief. Hopefully you may intend to continue most of these habits and so you don't really see how you can celebrate your success, since that emotional attachment to food is likely to be well behind you.

Remember when you might have eaten because you were happy or sad, stressed or excited? Remember when you may have eaten and not even realised what or how much you were eating?

Take a look at this list below and compare the 'before' with 'now'. What differences are there for you?

- Chewing
- Focusing on meals without distraction
- Regular eating
- Energy levels
- Food choices
- Mood swings
- Confidence

- Understanding of the body's reaction to food
- Sleep
- Muscle condition
- Complexion
- General appearance
- Fitness
- Your goals

Your final checkpoint

Don't delay with your final checkpoint. Turn to page 50 or 51 and compare your changes. I have seen so many become quite blasé with their achievement and so don't measure or record their changes and progress. Months down the line they always regret this. Knowing and seeing how far you've come is such a huge motivator in wanting to hang on to what you've earned yourself.

So, to make sure you really know how far you've come:

Measure yourself As before, waist, chest and hips. Arms and thighs too if you did originally. Compare it to your previous measurements.

Weigh yourself Compare it to your pre *Tidy the Temple* weight. If you used a fat monitor, now is your big day to take your second reading.

Take photos Don't skip this bit. You'll be an inspiration to yourself! Same positions, same place, same distance from the camera, same clothes and ideally the same lighting.

Look at your original goals Look at any of the amendments you made along the way. Did you reach them? And if not, knowing all you know now, were they realistic within this time span? What goals would you set out for yourself now?

PERSONAL POINT

I once kept my 'clean out' going for seven weeks without interruption. I'd just run a *Tidy the Temple* course and following that I was shooting some fitness DVDs.

I'd kept going as I needed to keep my energy levels good for repeated 'takes' and I didn't fancy feeling bloated while demonstrating exercises for a 'flat tummy'! I was after all, about to be immortalised on to film. After the shoot I flew to meet my family in Italy; Italy, of all places, the land of flavour and ice cream.

The first couple of days went ok and apart from a bit of bloating and feeling dopey, I thought I'd got away with any reactions to the change of diet.

Then by the third day the water retention was obvious and the tightness of it was making me feel stiff.

I went for a run in a hopeless attempt to shed the excess. Instead of galloping along like a gazelle as I'd become used to, I thundered along, heavy limbed with my water-logged flesh aching. It actually mildly hurt as it blobbed around.

It was a familiar feeling to post Caesarean and knee operations; lots of excess, goodness knows what kind of water hoarding in the cells. On top of this, my joints ached. This, I thought, is a taste of the future if I don't get a lifetime grip on my love for the Italian sweet trolley …

A word of warning, as explained in the 'Moving on from here' chapter (page 145). A celebratory drink, meal or treat that goes quite outside your recent eating habits may not leave you feeling so great. In fact, it will certainly be a reminder of how clean you have become over this time.

The reactions can vary from feeling drowsy to feeling quite unwell. Sore throats, headaches, feeling bloated, a churning stomach or alcohol going straight to your head, are just some of the remarks people have made. Don't worry though, this is only a sign that your body is letting you know it disagrees with this substance, whereas before you couldn't hear or heed its warning!

REMEMBER

Check you have done all the self tests that are on Day 27's message.

Keep up the good habits

Mostly people want to carry on with their new ways and going back to old habits leaves them feeling lousy. For many, not drinking alcohol for as long as 28 days is a first since puberty! Yet somehow that glass of wine that they thought they would so enjoy, just doesn't taste the same.

This just goes to show how tuned our palate becomes with our habits. Give it lots of enhanced flavour and sweeteners and it loses its touch for subtle tastes. Now after all this time of non-enhanced food and drinks, it goes back to having more acute taste – just like a baby.

You are back in neutral.

ACID/ALKALINE ROUGH GUIDE

ACID FORMING FOODS

Alcohol

Asparagus

Cheese (hard)

Cocoa

Coffee

Cornstarch

Egg yolks

Fish

Flour products (pasta, bread etc.)

Maple syrup

Meat

Milk and dairy

Molasses

Mustard

Noodles

Oatmeal

Oats

Offal

Pickles

Pork

Refined cereal

Sodas

Sweeteners

Wheat

White rice

Drugs, stress, anger, jealousy, fatigue!

LESS ACIDIC

Banana

Brown rice and basmati

Buckwheat

Cheese (soft)

Chickpeas

Cranberries

Fish

Legumes (e.g. beans, peas and lentils)

Onions

Plums

Prunes

Pulses

Rice milk

Seeds

Soy sauce

Spelt

Wholewheat

NEUTRAL

Butter cream

Plain yoghurt

Raw milk

Vegetable oil

ALKALINE AND SLIGHTLY ALKALINE FORMING FOODS:

Almonds

Apples

Artichokes

Asparagus

Aubergines

Avocados

Barley grass

Brussel sprouts

Celery

Cherries

Chestnuts

Coconuts

Corn

Courgettes

Cucumbers

Dates

Egg whites

Endives

Figs

Fruits

Garlic

Goat's milk

Grapefruits

Grapes

Greens

Honey

Leeks

Lemons

Limes

Melons

Millet

Miso

Mushrooms

Olives and olive oil

Oranges

Papaya

Parsnips

Peaches

Pears

Peas

Pineapple

Potatoes

Pumpkin

Quince

Quinoa

Raisins

Rhubarb

Sea vegetables

Sesame

Soya products

Tomatoes

Vegetables

Watermelons

Wheat grass

Peace, love and kindness!

This is a rough guide and you may find references that differ from one another. For instance, grapefruits, limes and peppers are just a few that are considered alkaline in some health guides, yet acidic according to Chinese medicine.

EXERCISE ROUTINES
For All Levels

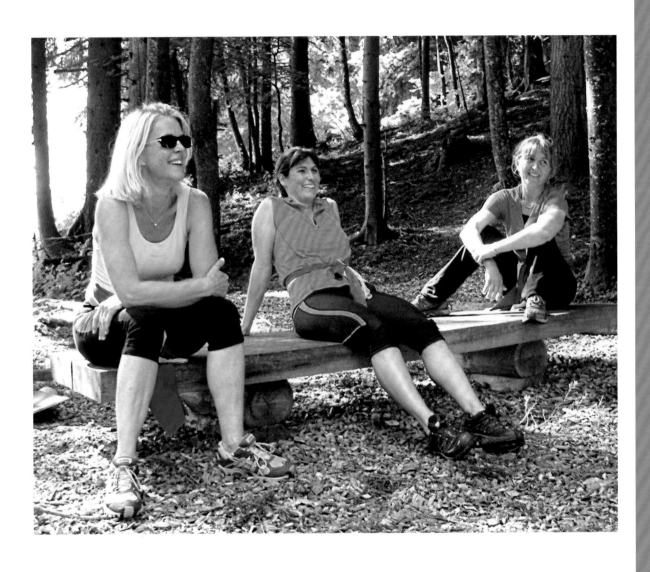

Starter's Exercises

Turn to page 25 for more information about what you will need before starting.

Warm up

1. Knee Lifts

8 steady paced knee lifts on each leg. Get the arms moving too.

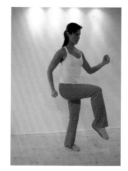 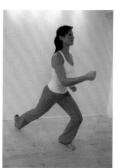

2. Punches

8 slow punches each side. Rotate waist and hips. Knees bend and extend.

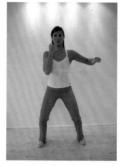 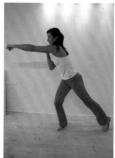

3. Step Ups

Stairs or a sturdy ledge will do fine. Slow stepping up and down. 10 each side.

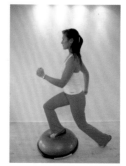 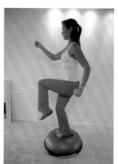

4. Swing Through

Bend from the knees and flex from the hips, keep the back straight and allow the weight to give you momentum to swing low and high. 8 each side.

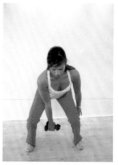 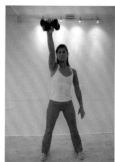

Starter's Exercises Workout

These 25 exercises will take approximately 12 minutes when you get used to the routine. Move swiftly between each exercise so as to keep the heart rate varied. Mostly, it is every other exercise which is designed to raise the heart rate. Some exercises may feel quite hard at first to repeat as many times as recommended. Just work towards this over time.

Pay attention to doing each movement as the photographs illustrate and read the points.

1. Clean and Press *Areas worked: shoulders, legs, buttocks.*

Weights in each hand, feet slightly apart, raise the weights up sideways to shoulder height, make sure the elbows are slightly bent and the thumbs tilt forward and downwards, and then lower. Keep posture straight throughout.

Repeat 15–20 times or for 30 seconds.

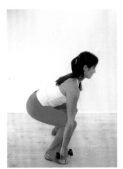 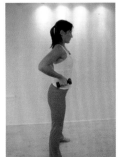 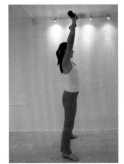

2. Shoulder Raise *Areas worked: top middle part of the shoulders.*

Weights in each hand, feet hip distance apart, knees bent, spine long and straight. Straighten the legs while raising weights to side at rib height then push upwards, straightening the arms. Come down through the same sequence.

Repeat 12 times. Steady speed.

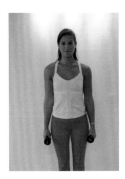 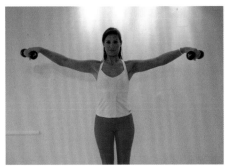

3. Rotating Pick Ups *Areas worked: shoulders, legs, buttocks and obliques.*

Similar to exercise 1 but lock the weights together and place them to the side of the outer left leg. Lift them up with a straight spine, using leg power to straighten the legs, then arms above the head and rotate down to the right side. Draw the tummy in to help keep the back strong and straight.

Repeat 12–15 repetitions or for 30 seconds.

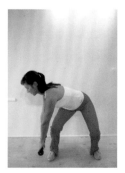 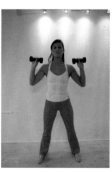 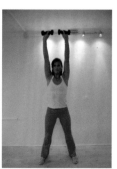 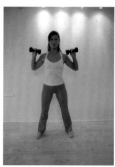 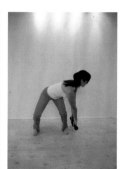

4. Kick Backs *Areas worked: backs of arms, triceps.*

With a weight in each hand elbows high, place the weights by the ribs. Keep knees bent, hinge forward from the hips with the spine straight and maintain this posture throughout the exercise. Extend the arms straight behind keeping them high, nearly locking out the elbow and return to the elbow bend each time.

Repeat 20–30 times or for 30 seconds.

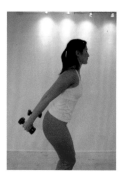 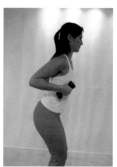

5. Lift and Rise *Areas worked: upper and lower legs, buttocks, biceps, back.*

With a weight in each hand, feet hip distance apart, squat down hinging from the knees and hips while looking forward. Pull up the weights swiftly as you straighten up and rise on your toes, tucking the weights nearly to the underarm. Drop down to the starting position and rise up again quickly.

Repeat 12–15 times or for 30 seconds.

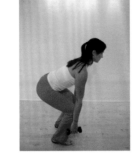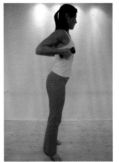

6. One-Legged Bicep Curls *Areas worked: biceps and midsection, core.*

Standing on one leg with the weight in the hand, arm straight, bend the elbow and curl the weight up towards you slowly and controlled. Standing on one leg ensures all the work goes into the bicep.

Repeat for 20 plus times or for 30 seconds.

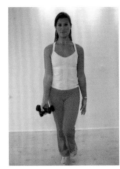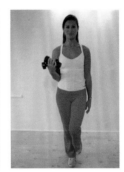

7 & 8. Wood Chops *Areas worked: obliques, legs, shoulders.*

Lock weights together and hold them up high to the right side. Take most of your balance on the right leg. As if swinging an axe, chop the weights down diagonally to the lower left side. Make sure the back is long and straight and you only bend in the knees and hips. Stop and hold a split second as you pass the knee. Swing back up, stopping sharply up top again. Make sure you control the movement rather than allowing the weight's momentum to swing and twist you around.

Repeat 10 times on each side.

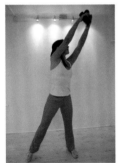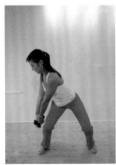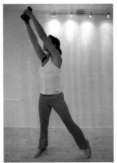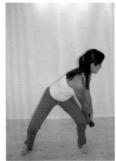

9 . One-Legged Bicep Curls *Areas worked: biceps and midsection, core.*

Standing on one leg with the weight in the opposite hand, arm straight, bend the elbow and curl the weight up towards you slowly and controlled. Standing on one leg ensures all the work goes into the bicep.

Repeat for 20 plus times or for 30 seconds.

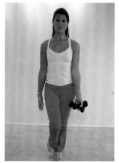 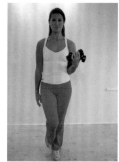

10. Swing Through and Press *Areas worked: legs, shoulders.*

With both weights locked together, squat down with arms hanging straight down holding the weights. Keep looking forward and swing the weights up to the chest, bending the arms. Then straighten the arms upwards above the head. Return by bringing the hands back to the chest and then swing down between the legs.

Repeat 12 times.

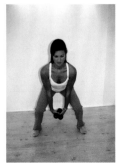 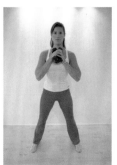 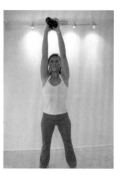 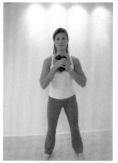 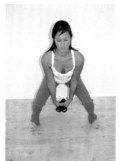

11. Wide Row *Areas worked: back.*

With a weight in each hand, bend forward from the hips with a straight spine and the knees bent. Allow the arms to hang straight down and then, bending the elbows, lift the weights to waist level. Keep the elbows wide and squeeze the shoulder blades together as you lift the weights. Keep it slow and controlled with good posture.

Repeat 20 times or for 30 seconds.

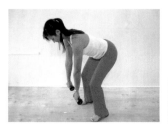 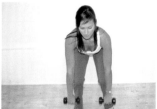 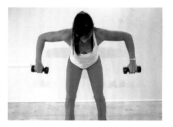

12. Squat and Kick *Areas worked: legs, buttocks.*

Without weights, place the feet apart and get into a good squat position, a little wider than normal. Straighten the legs, lift up the left leg and kick it out sideways. Return to the squat, lift the right leg out and kick.

Repeat 20 alternating sides.

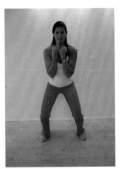 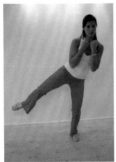 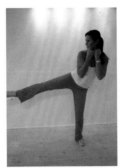

13. Narrow Squats *Areas worked: legs, buttocks.*

Narrow squats can soften the line of the thigh muscle and make more of a feminine sweep than a bulky one. Holding the weights and with the feet neatly together, bend from the hips and knees. If you find it restrictive, you may find it easier to put something beneath the heels (a couple of magazines or a folded mat). This enables more depth to the bend. Take it slow to start and then change the pace, i.e. slowly down, fast up and fast down, slowly up.

Repeat 20–25 times.

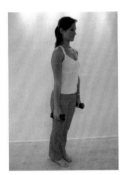 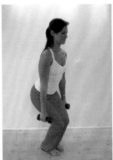

14. Side Lunge Jumps *Areas worked: legs, buttocks.*

With the left leg out to the side and the right leg bent with body weight and hands on it, jump up high and switch legs in the air, landing on the left leg. Keep bending and straightening your knees to absorb the bounce and power. Make sure the knees are aligned with the toes.

Repeat 20 times.

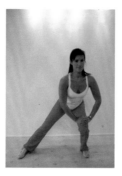 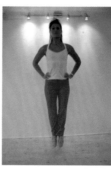 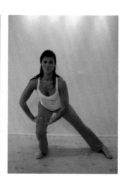

15. Tricep Dips *Areas worked: backs of arms, triceps.*

As if about to sit, on the floor, keep the weight between hands and feet only. Make sure the fingers turn in the direction of the backside. Keep the hands quite close together. Bend the elbows and lower towards the floor. Make sure that it is your elbows that are bending and not just your hips lifting up and down.

Aim for 20 times or 30 seconds.

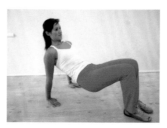 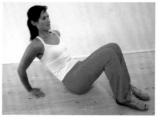

16. Narrow Star Jump *Areas worked: legs, buttocks.*

Starting with feet together and knees bent, like a narrow squat, jump upwards while splitting the legs and opening the arms out. Land back in the narrow squat.

Repeat 20 times.

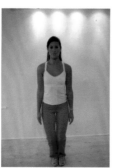 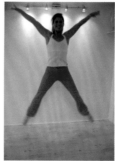

17. Kneeling Shoulder Press *Areas worked: shoulders and upper back.*

Kneeling upright on the mat (with the backside off the heels), take the weights in each hand and position them squarely at shoulder height. Push the weights upwards and touch them together above the head as if making a pyramid shape. Try to relax the shoulders and keep them low.

Repeat 20–25 times.

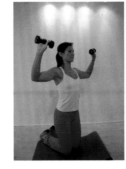 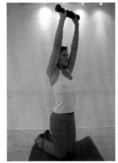

18. Clapping Feet Squat Jumps *Areas worked: legs, buttocks.*

Starting in a squat position with feet hip distance apart, hands on hips, jump upwards and snap the feet together before landing back in the squat again.

Repeat 20 times or for 30 seconds.

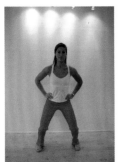 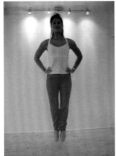 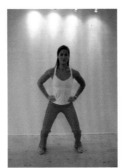

19 & 20. Single-Legged Squats *Areas worked: legs, outer thigh, balance and coordination.*

Stand on the left leg, with the arms out to the side and the other leg just off the ground. Squat down bending only from the knee and hip. Take it slowly and try to keep the back as straight as possible. Bringing the arms in for each bend may help with balance. Stay on this side for 12 repetitions and then switch sides.

Repeat 12 times each side.

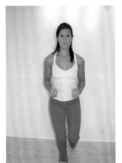 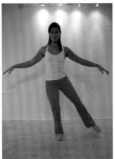 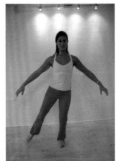 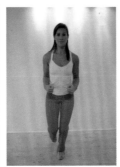

21 & 22. Oblique Hold *Areas worked: side and lower back, obliques.*

Lying on the left side on the mat, bend the elbow beneath for support. Make sure it is well beneath the shoulder joint and in line with it. Bend the underneath leg (the left) with the foot placed behind for further support. Now push up the hips, lifting them off the floor, hold them here, elevated for 10 counts. Then touch the hip down and lift again for 8 times. If it feels too easy, extend the underneath leg and position it slightly behind the top leg.

Repeat both sides 8 times.

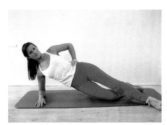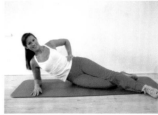

23. Sit-ups with Leg Raise *Areas worked: midsection.*

Lying on the back on the mat, lift the legs up and hold them squarely to the floor and your midsection; knees and hips bent at right angles. Hold the hands behind the head and relax and flatten the tummy. Think about the belly button sinking towards the spine. Breathe in then sit up just lifting the head and shoulders off the floor and exhale the breath. Breathe out as you come up and in as you come down. Keep it slow and controlled.

Repetitions 10–20 times or for 30 seconds. If you have a Swiss Ball, these next two exercises will really work the midsection just that bit more.

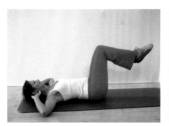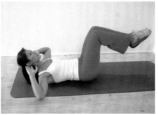

24. Elbows on Ball Hold and Roll *Areas worked: midsection, transversus, abdominals, lower back.*

If you have a ball, try these exercises too. Kneeling on the mat, place the elbows on the ball. Make sure the face is directly over the ball and over the hands, this makes the exercise more achievable and comfortable. Straighten out the body so that it is pencil straight from head to knees. You may already find the midsection is working in this position but if you wish to make it more intense, lift the knees off the mat and straighten the legs. Hold the position for 8 counts. Then very slightly, roll the ball away from you for 4 centimetres and pull it back.

Try this 5 times. Relax and repeat.

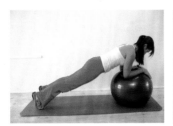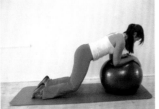

25. Feet on Ball Pulls *Areas worked: midsection, transversus, abdominals.*

With the hands on the floor, get the lower leg on to the ball. Walk away from the ball on the hands until the lower shin and upper side of the foot is resting on top of the ball. Widen the hands. With a very straight back, draw the knees towards the chest and then roll the ball back again. Ensure the back doesn't hyper extend or go banana shaped. Keep it steady and in good balance and control.

Repeat approximately 8 times.

Turn to page 127 and 128 for a short stretch sequence.

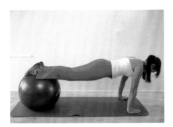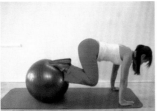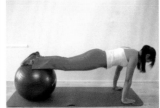

Intermediate Workout

Turn to page 25 for information on equipment needed.

Warm up

Just to get the body and back well mobilised, go through these following warm up exercises with about 8–10 repetitions of each movement.

1. Rotate round to one side and gently punch behind and high. Return to the front with the hands held to the shoulders. Rotate and punch lightly behind and high on the other side. Repeat about 10 times.

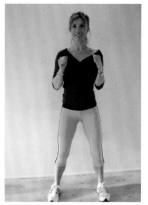 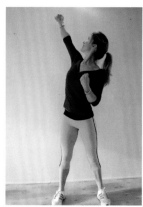 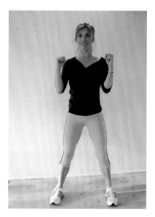 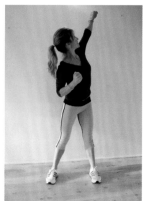

2. Bend both legs and reach to one side. Make sure to pull the underneath arm across and in the opposite direction from the bend. Come back to an upright position with the legs straight. Bend the knees and reach to the other side pulling the underneath arm away again. Repeat about 10 times.

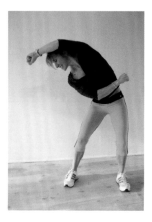 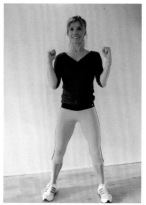 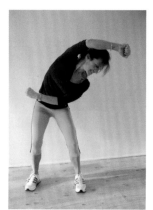

3. Bend both knees, reach low and forward with one hand to touch the floor in front. Switch arms and repeat on the other side.

Repeat about 8 times.

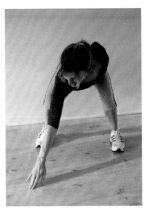 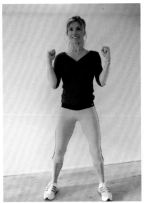 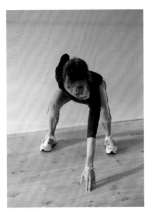

4. Bend both knees and touch the floor to the side. Allow the back to take a natural bend and twist.

Repeat 8 times.

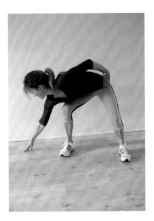 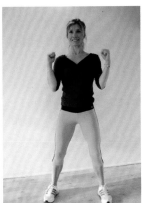 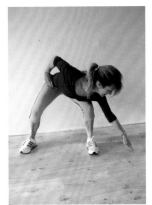

Exercises *Intermediate Workout*

1. Swing Through *Areas worked: legs, shoulders.*

With both weights locked together, squat down with the arms hanging straight down, keep looking forward while swinging the weights upwards above the head. Return by bringing the weights between the legs.

Repeat 12 times.

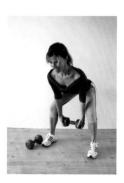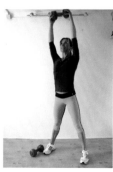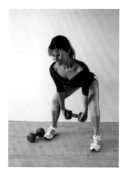

2. Side Circles *Areas worked: top and middle part of the shoulders.*

With a weight in each hand and feet slightly apart, raise the weights up sideways to shoulder height, make sure the elbows are slightly bent and the thumbs tilt forward and downwards. Make forward circular movements returning back to the side position with each circle. Keep posture straight throughout.

Repeat 12–15 times.

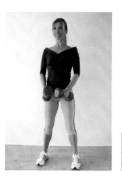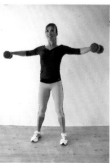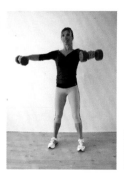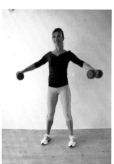

3. Swing Round *Areas worked: shoulders, arms, midsection.*

With both hands, hold each end of one weight. Push the weight out sideways at waist level, swing it round with the arms straight to the other side and pull it inwards. Push outwards from that side and swing straight to the other side.

Repeat 16 times.

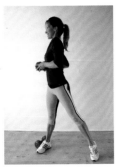 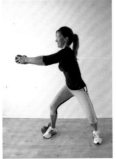 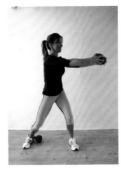 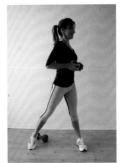

4. Shoulder Side Raises *Areas worked: top and middle part of the shoulders.*

With a weight in each hand and feet slightly apart, raise the weights up sideways to shoulder height, make sure the elbows are slightly bent and the thumbs tilt forward and downwards. Then lower back to the start position. Keep posture straight throughout.

Repeat 15–20 times or for 30 seconds.

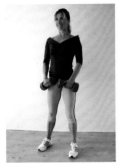 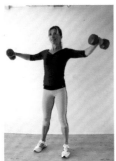 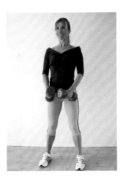

5. Boxing Feet *Areas worked: legs, agility.*

Step and dash from side to side, joining the feet with each step sideways at a fast pace.

Repeat for 30 seconds.

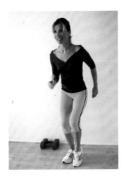 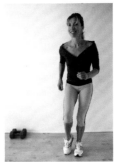

6. Shoulder Press *Areas worked: shoulders, upper back.*

Standing upright with feet apart, take the weights in each hand and position them squarely at shoulder height. Push the weights upwards and touch them together above the head as if making a pyramid shape. Try to relax the shoulders and keep them low. Bring the weights back down to the start position.

Repeat 20–25 times.

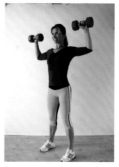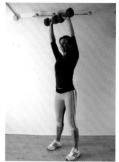

7 & 8. Wood Chops *Areas worked: midsection, obliques, shoulders.*

Lock weights together and hold them up high to the right side. Take most of your balance on the right leg. As if swinging an axe, chop the weights down diagonally to the lower left side. Make sure the back is long and straight and the only bend is in the knees and hips. Stop and hold a split second as you pass the knee. Swing back up stopping sharply at the top again. Make sure you control the movement rather than allowing the weights' momentum to swing and twist you around

Repeat both sides 8 times.

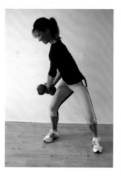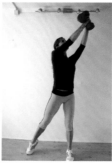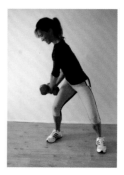

9. Squats *Areas worked: legs, buttocks.*

Holding the weights and with the feet hip distance apart, bend from the hips and knees. Take 6 slow squats to start, 3 seconds down, 3 seconds up. Then change the pace and take 6 fast, still keeping the positions correct. Follow with 6 at a normal speed.

Repeat 18 times.

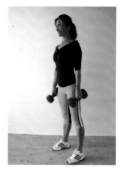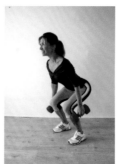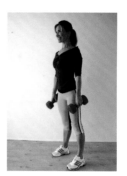

10 & 11. Single Swing *Areas worked: legs, buttocks, shoulder.*

With the feet hip distance apart, hold a weight in one hand and swing the weight high and low in front of you, with a deep bend as you lower. Keep the arm and back straight while just hinging from the knees and hips to bend as you lower the weight.

Repeat both sides 8 times.

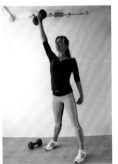 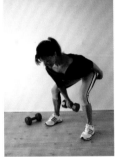 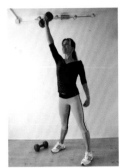

12 & 13. Front Lunge *Areas worked: Legs, backside.*

Holding a weight in each hand, step forward and lunge, keeping the knee and hip bent at 90 degrees. Pay attention to the upper body sitting centrally and upright in the lunge. Keep the weight on this front foot and push up to straight legs using the power from the front leg. Keep the front foot in the same position throughout the exercise.

Stay on the same side for 12–15 repetitions, then repeat on the other side.

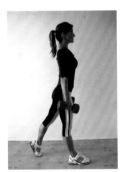 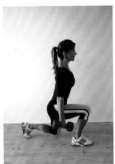 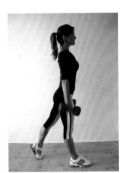

14. Swing Through and Press *Areas worked: legs, shoulders.*

Taking one heavy weight or with both weights locked together, squat down with arms hanging straight down, keep looking forward while swinging the weights up to the chest, bending the arms, then straightening the arms upwards above the head. Return by bringing the hands back to the chest and then swing down between the legs.

Repeat 12 times.

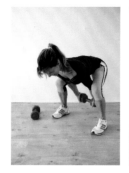 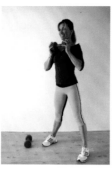 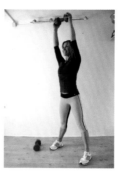 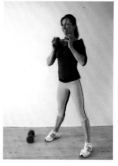 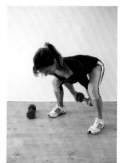

15. Bicep Curls and Hold *Areas worked: tops of arms, biceps.*

Standing with legs hip distance apart and a weight in each hand, bend the elbow and curl the weight up towards you slowly and with control.

Repeat 15 times and then hold in the halfway position for 10 seconds. Then make 8 mini curls from this halfway position. Finish with 6 full curls.

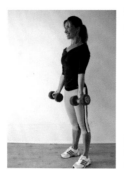 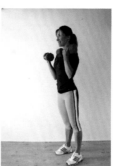 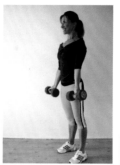 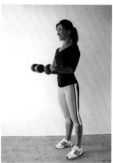

16. Sporty Feet *Areas worked: agility and cardio system.*

With the feet apart and weight mostly on the ball of the foot, stride across the other leg as if dashing about in a sport. Staying on the same side, bounce back and forth, keeping nice and agile while driving the arms with the action.

Repeat 10 times on each side.

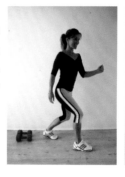 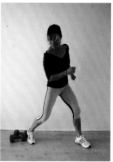

17. Tricep Kick Backs *Areas worked: backs of arms, triceps.*

With a weight in each hand, the elbows high, place the weights by the ribs with the palms inwards. Keep the knees bent and hinge forward from the hips with the spine straight, maintain this posture throughout the exercise. Still with the palms facing inwards, extend the arms straight behind keeping them high, nearly locking out the elbow. Return to the start position.

Repeat 20 times or for 30 seconds.

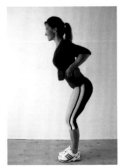 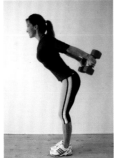 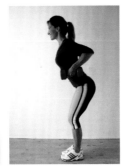

18. Side Lunge Jumps *Areas worked: legs, buttocks.*

With the left leg out to the side and the right leg bent with weight and hands on it, jump up high and switch legs in the air, landing on the left leg. Keep jumping and switching sides. Make sure your knees bend and straighten to absorb the bounce and power. Also make sure the knees are aligned with the toes.

Repeat 20 times.

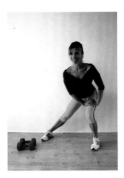 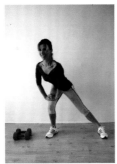 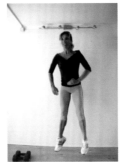

19. Tricep Dips *Areas worked: backs of arms, triceps.*

As if about to sit on the floor, hold your weight between hands and feet only. Make sure the fingers turn in the direction of the backside. Keep the hands quite close together. Bend the elbows and lower towards the floor. Come back to the start position. Make sure that it is your elbows that are bending and not just your hips lifting up and down.

Repeat 20 times or for 30 seconds.

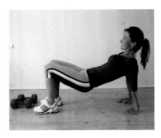 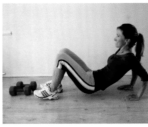 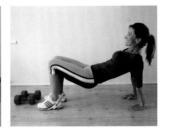

20. Clean and Rise *Areas Worked: legs, lower and upper back, biceps.*

With toes pointing forwards and feet hip distance apart, take a weight in each hand and bend down with the weights touching the floor. Keep the spine long and eyes looking ahead. Power yourself up on to the toes with speed, straightening the legs and snapping the weights upwards to under the armpit. Keep the elbows tight behind. Keep balance and drop back down to the start position.

Repeat 15 times or for 30 seconds.

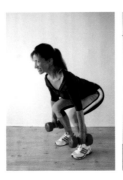 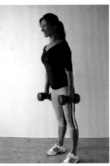 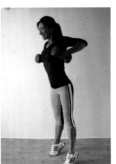 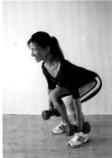

21. Wide Pull *Areas worked: back, biceps.*

With a weight in each hand, bend forward from the hips with a straight spine, keeping the knees bent. Allow the arms to hang straight down with the knuckles facing away from you. Then bend the elbows and lift the weights up to waist level. Keep the elbows wide and squeeze the shoulder blades together as you lift the weights. Bring them back to start position. Keep it slow and controlled with good posture.

Repeat 20 times or for 30 seconds.

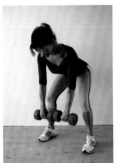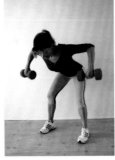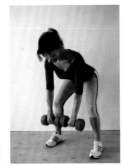

22. Cross Squat Jumps *Areas worked: legs, backside.*

Position the feet hip distance apart with the hands on hips. Jump upwards and land with the feet crossed over, jump up and cross them again landing with the other foot crossed in front. Jump up again and land with them apart as the starting position. Keep this well-paced with powerful jumps.

Repeat for 30 seconds.

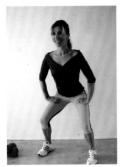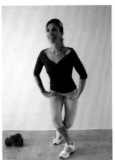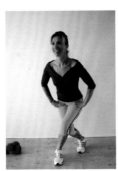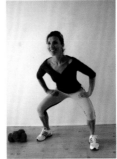

23. Press-ups *Areas worked: front shoulder, chest.*

On all fours, place the hands slightly wider than shoulder width on the floor, fingers forward. Drop the knees on the mat and make sure the body line from head to heel is straight without bends or dips. Lower the chest and nose to the floor keeping the same straight line and push up again. If you have the force, lift the knees up and straighten the legs.

Repeat for 20 seconds.

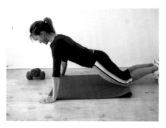 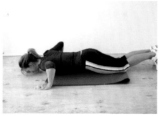 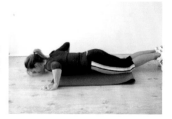

24. Jumping Squats *Areas worked: legs, buttocks.*

Feet positioned in the squat position, with arms by the sides, bend deep into the squat and power jump upwards. Keep the hands on the hips or swing them forward to assist the elevation. Land in a good bend and jump again.

Repeat 10–12 times.

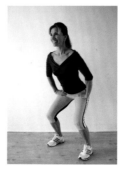 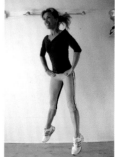

25. Spiderman Press-ups *Areas worked: chest, front shoulder.*

On all fours, tuck the toes under and position the left leg further forward than the right. Now slide the left hand up higher than the right as if making a Spiderman shape. Press down, lowering the chest and nose to the floor 5 or 6 times before switching leg and hand position over.

Repeat 10–12 in total.

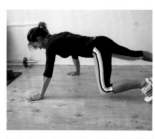 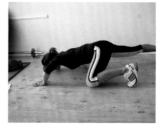

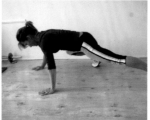 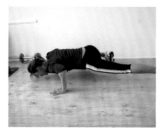

26. Scissor Sit-ups *Areas worked: abdominals, midsection.*

Lying on the mat on the back, bend the knees up to a 90 degree angle and hold the hands gently behind the neck. Take a breath in and, as you exhale, lift the head and shoulders off the floor while straightening the legs into a scissor split. To avoid back discomfort, make sure the legs are no lower than 45 degrees. As you breathe in, come back to the start position with the head back on the floor. Repeat the other side and scissor split with the other leg leading. With each sit-up and split, slightly twist the torso towards the higher leg.

Repeat 12–16 times.

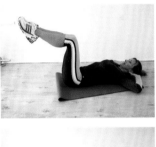 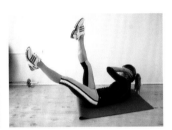

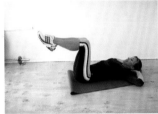 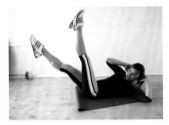

27. Oblique Hold *Areas worked: side and lower back, obliques.*

Lying on the left side on the mat, bend the elbow beneath for support. Make sure it is well beneath the shoulder joint and in line with it. Both legs are straight but place the higher one with the foot slightly further forward than the underneath foot (to make it easier bend the underneath leg with the foot placed behind). Now push up the hips, lifting them off the floor, hold them here, elevated for 10 counts. Then touch the hip down and lift again for 8 times.

Repeat on the other side. Hold for 10 counts. Raise hips up and down 8 times.

Turn to pages 127 and 128 for a short stretch sequence.

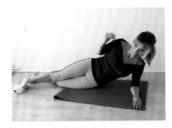 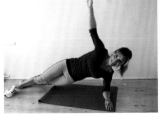

Experienced Exerciser's Workout

Turn to page 25 for information on equipment needed.

Warm up

Just to get the body mobilised, go through these following warm up exercises with about 6–8 repetitions of each movement.

1. Transfer the weight to one side and alternately curl the leg behind.

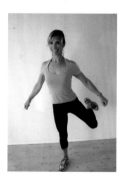 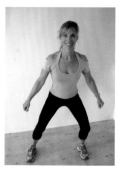 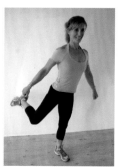

2. Standing on one leg, raise the other knee high and touch back down behind between each knee raise. Drive the arms well in opposition to the leg lift.

Repeat about 8 times on each side.

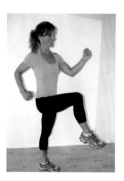 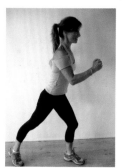

3. Repeat the knee adding an outward circular movement to mobilise the hip joint.

Repeat about 8 times on each side.

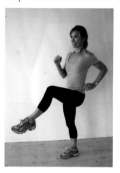 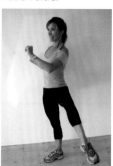 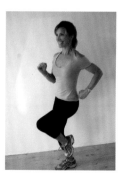

Exercises *Experienced Exerciser's Workout*

1. Wood Chops *Areas worked: midsection, obliques, shoulders.*

Lock weights together and hold them up high to the right side. Take most of your balance on the right leg. As if swinging an axe, chop the weights down diagonally to the lower left side. Make sure the back is long and straight and you only bend in the knees and hips. Stop and hold a split second as you pass the knee. Swing back up stopping sharply at the top again. Make sure you control the movement rather than allowing the weights' momentum to swing and twist you around.

Repeat 8 on one side before changing to the other side.

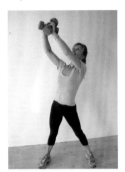 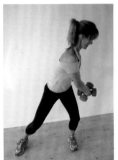

2. Kneeling Press *Areas worked: shoulders, upper back.*

Kneeling upright on the mat (with the backside off the heels), take the weights in each hand and position them squarely at shoulder height. Push the weights upwards and touch them together above the head as if making a pyramid shape. Try to relax the shoulders and keep them low. Bring the weights back down to the start position.

Repeat 20–25 times.

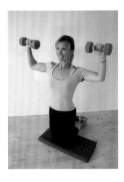 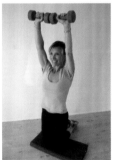

3. Swing Through and Press *Areas worked: legs, shoulders.*

With both weights locked together, squat down with arms hanging straight down, keep looking forward while swinging the weights up to the chest, bending the arms, then straightening the arms upwards above the head. Return by bringing the hands back to the chest and then swinging down between the legs.

Repeat 12 times.

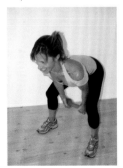 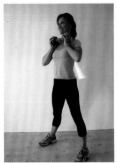 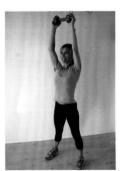 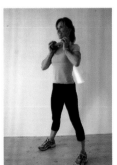 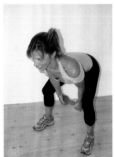

4. Speed Squats *Areas worked: legs, buttocks.*

With the feet hip distance apart and keeping the back straight, bend from the hips and knees. Take 8 bends slowly to start, then 8 very fast, still keeping the correct movement, followed by 8 very slow squats.

Repeat 24 times in total.

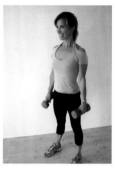 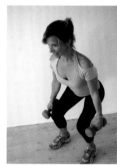

5. Side Raises and Bounces *Areas worked: top and middle part of the shoulders.*

With a weight in each hand and feet slightly apart, raise the weights up sideways to shoulder height, make sure the elbows are slightly bent and the thumbs tilt forward and downwards. Then lower back to the start position. Keep posture straight throughout.

Repeat 20 times and then straight into the following exercise.

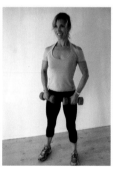 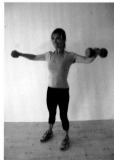 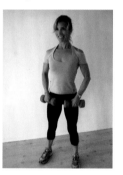

6. Shoulder Raises

Holding the weights out to the side, make mini moves, lifting and lowering them fractionally.

Repeat 6–10 repetitions then repeat the full raises up and down 4 more times.

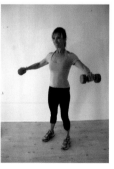 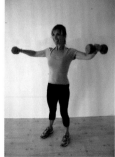

7. Sporty Feet *Areas worked: agility and cardio sytem.*

With the feet apart and weight mostly on the ball of the foot, softly stride across the other leg as if dashing about in a sport. Staying on the same side, bounce back and forth, keeping nice and agile while driving the arms with the action.

Repeat 10 times on each side.

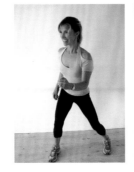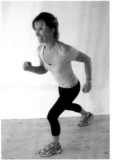

8. Shoulder Press on Hands *Areas worked: shoulders, arms, chest.*

With the hands shoulder width apart on the floor, fingers pointing forwards, lift the backside high and put most of your body weight on to your hands. Try to make a V-shape but bend the knees if flexibility is restricting you. Bend the elbows and lower the head down until it touches the floor then push up to the start position.

Repeat as many times as you are able in 30 seconds.

WARNING: This is quite hard-core! But to make it even harder, raise one leg high and transfer more weight on to the hands.

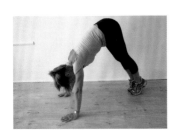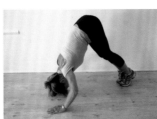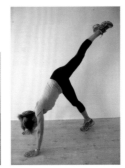

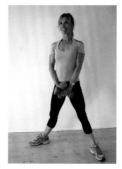
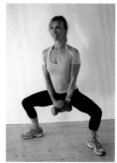

9. Wide Plié Squats *Areas worked: legs, inner thigh, lower backside.*

Hold both weights locked together. With the feet wide and turned out as if in a ballet stance, bend the knees nice and wide, keeping them in line with the toes. Keep the back up straight and bend quite low. Take these bends slowly and with precision. Squeeze and lift the leg and backside muscles during the lowering and rising movement.

Repeat 20 times before moving straight on to the following variation.

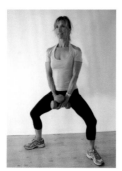
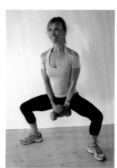

10. Wide Plié Mini Squats

Holding the same position without a rest, stay low in the bend and make small bounces up and down, keep the muscles tight.

Repeat 8 bounces and then 4 full bends again.
Repeat twice.

11. Wide Plié Squats with Heel Lift

Still down in that position, raise one heel and lower down and up before switching to raise the other heel. Keep alternating heel raises.

Repeat 8 times and finish with 2 full bends.

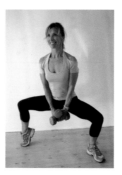
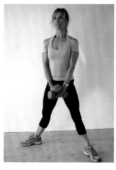
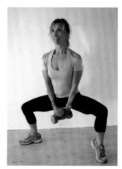

12. Clean and Rise *Areas Worked: legs, lower and upper back, biceps.*

With toes pointing forwards and feet hip distance apart, take a weight in each hand and bend down with the weights touching the floor. Keep the spine long and eyes looking ahead. Power yourself up on to the toes with speed, straightening the legs and snapping the weights upwards to under the armpit. Keep the elbows tight behind. Keep balance and drop back down to the start position.

Repeat 15–20 times or for 30 seconds.

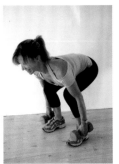 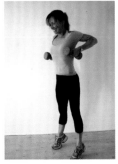 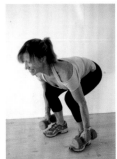

13. Wide Pull *Areas worked: back, biceps.*

With a weight in each hand, bend forward from the hips with a straight spine and the knees bent. Allow the arms to hang straight down with the knuckles facing away from you. Then bend the elbows and lift the weights up to waist level. Keep the elbows wide and squeeze the shoulder blades together as you lift the weights. Bring them back to the start position. Keep it slow and controlled with good posture.

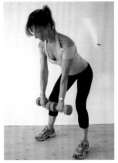 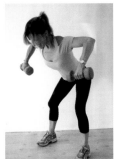

Repeat 20 times or for 30 seconds.

14 & 15. Lunge and Press *Areas worked: legs, backside, shoulders, midsection.*

Holding the weight in one hand, step forward and lunge down while pushing the weight upwards, above the shoulder. Return the weight and leg back to the starting position. Stay on the same side keeping it steady and well executed.

Repeat both sides 12 times.

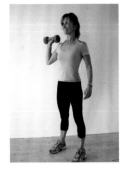 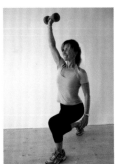 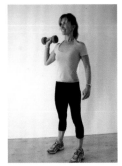

16 & 17. Single Arm Row *Areas worked: back, biceps.*

With feet slightly apart, knees softly bent, hinge forward from the hips with a straight back. Take one heavy weight or holding both weights locked together in one hand, allow the arm to hang down straight. Pull it up to the armpit keeping the elbow close to the ribs. Lower the weights back down. Throughout the exercise leave the other arm hanging and unsupported. This helps the midsection work more.

Repeat both sides 16–20 times.

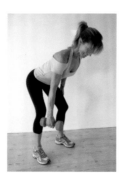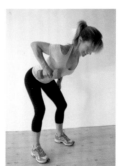

18. Star Jump *Areas worked: legs, buttocks.*

Start with feet together and knees bent, like a narrow squat, jump upwards while splitting the legs and opening the arms out. Land back in the narrow squat. Jump up and split straight away and keep momentum.

Repeat 20 times.

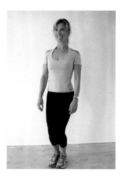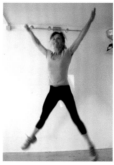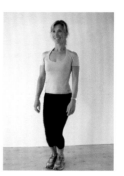

19. Tricep Kick Backs and Rotations *Areas worked: backs of arms, triceps.*

With a weight in each hand and the elbows high, place the weights by the ribs with the palms inwards. Keep the knees bent and hinge forward from the hips with the spine straight, maintain this posture throughout the exercise. Still with the palms facing inwards, extend the arms straight behind keeping them high, nearly locking out the elbow. Return to the start postion. Take 8 repetitions like this then change the angle of the hands by turning the thumb outwards, continue for 8. Lastly rotate the thumbs inwards and repeat for 8. See the photograph for these variations of hand positions.

Repeat 8 times with palms inwards, 8 times thumbs outwards, 8 times thumbs inwards.

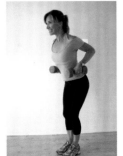 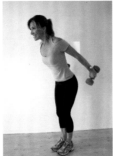 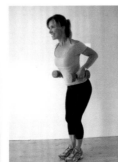 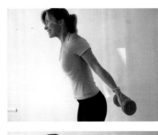 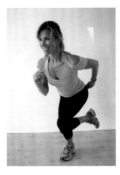

20 & 21. Single-Legged Squat *Areas worked: legs, outer thigh, balance and coordination.*

Stand on the left leg, with arms out to the side and the other leg just off the ground. Squat down, bending only from the knee and hip. Straighten back up to start position. Take it slowly and try to keep the back as straight as possible. Bringing the arms in for the bend may help with balance.

Repeat both sides 12–14 times.

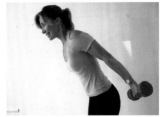 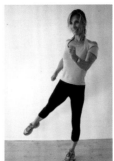

22. Side Lunge Jumps *Areas worked: legs, buttocks.*

With the left leg out to the side and the right leg bent with weight and hands on it, jump up high and switch legs in the air, landing on the left leg. Keep switching sides. Make sure your knees bend and straighten to absorb the bounce and power, make sure the knees are aligned with the toes.

Repeat 20 times.

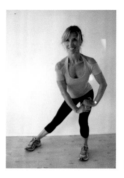 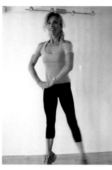 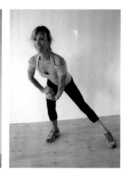

23. Tricep Dips *Areas worked: backs of arms, triceps.*

As if about to sit on the floor, hold your weight between hands and feet only. Make sure the fingers turn in the direction of the backside, keep the hands quite close together. Bend the elbows and lower towards the floor. Come back to the start position. Make sure that it is your elbows that are bending and not just your hips lifting up and down.

Aim for 20 times or 30 seconds. To increase the intensity lift one arm.

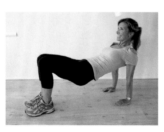 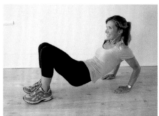 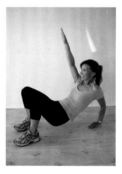

24. Clapping Squat Jumps *Areas worked: legs, buttocks.*

Starting in a squat position, with feet hip distance apart, power jump up and clap the feet together, landing back in the squat. Keep the hands on the hips. Make sure knees are over the toes with each landing and that the bend for the jump comes only from the knees and hips.

Repeat 20 times.

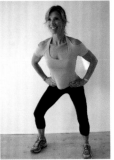
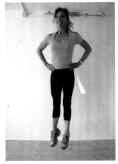
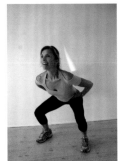

25. Press-ups *Areas worked: front shoulder, chest.*

On all fours, place the hands slightly wider than shoulder width on the floor, fingers forward. Tuck the toes under, straighten the legs and make sure the body line from head to heel is straight without bends or dips. Lower the chest and nose to the floor keeping the same straight line and push up again. Start like this and then drop the knees to the floor as soon as you need to make the last repetitions easier.

Repeat for 30 seconds.

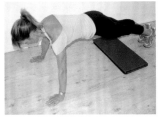
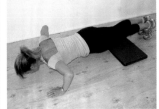
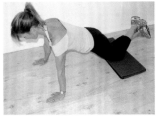
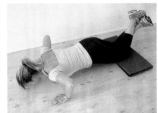

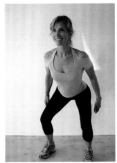
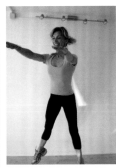

26. Squat Jumps *Areas worked: legs, buttocks.*

Feet positioned in the squat position, with arms by the sides, bend deep into the squat and with lots of power jump up, swinging the arms forward. Land in a good bend with the arms back by the sides.

Repeat 20 times.

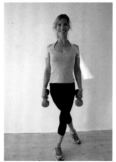
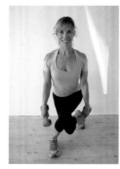

27 & 28. Curtsy *Areas worked: legs, outer and back of thigh, backside.*

Holding a weight in each hand, tuck one leg behind the other. Keep all the weight on the front leg and lower down sitting slightly towards the supporting foot. Keep the back upright and focus on the outer hip area. Come back up to the start position. Make sure the hips face forward throughout the movement and move slowly up and down.

Repeat both sides 12 times.

29. Spiderman Press-ups *Areas worked: chest, front shoulder.*

On all fours, tuck the toes under and position the left leg further forward than the right. Now slide the left hand up higher than the right as if making a Spidernan shape. Press down 6–8 times before switching leg and hand position over.

Repeat 12–16 times in total.

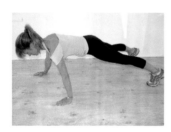
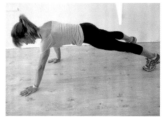
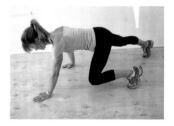

30. Squat Jump Turns *Areas worked: legs, buttocks.*

Feet positioned in the squat position, with arms by the sides, bend deep into the squat and power jump up, turning 180 degrees. Keep the hands on the hips. Land in a good bend and jump back round 180 degrees.

Repeat 14 times.

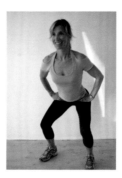
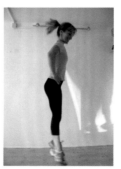
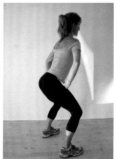

31. Plank and Variations *Areas worked: midsection, core.*

Lying facedown on a mat, propped up with the elbows, make sure the body line from head to heels is perfectly straight. The feet can be slightly apart. If the position brings lower back discomfort, raise the backside fractionally. Hold this position for 10 counts. Lower the knees to rest on the mat if it feels too strenuous.

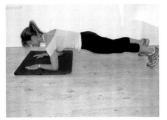 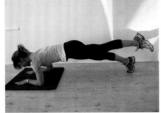 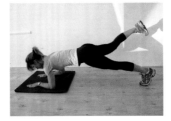

32. Knee Drops *Areas worked: midsection, core.*

Continuing from the plank position, lift one leg a few centimetres. Hold for 5 counts or more.

Change sides and repeat. Still maintaining the plank, widen the feet a fraction and, without moving anything other than the knees, bend the knees and touch the mat. Hold them a second and then straighten them as before.

Repeat 8 knee bends.

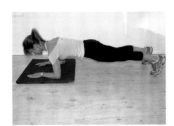 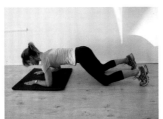

33. Paper Slides, Alternating *Areas worked: midsection, upper thigh, hip flexors.*

With two pieces of paper, put one beneath each foot and get on to all fours, creating a straight line like that of the Plank. Slide one leg inwards bending the knee towards the hips. Now switch and slide the other foot and knee up. Keep the feet central on the paper.

Repeat 20 times.

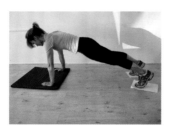 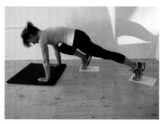 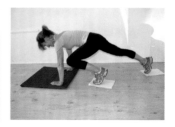

34. Paper Slides, both legs.

Continuing on from the previous exercise, draw both knees in at the same time and slide them back to start position.

Repeat 8 times.

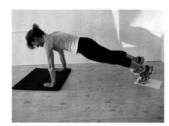 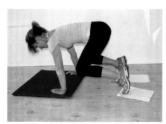 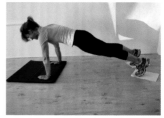

35. Crunches, knees raised *Areas worked: midsection.*

Lying on your back on a mat, place the fingers loosely behind the head. Lift the knees up and bend them so that the hips and knee joints are at 90 degree angles. Take a breath in and as you exhale, sit up and reach the arms out towards the straightened legs. Breathe in as you come back to the start position. Keep the movement slow and, with each out breath, ensure the stomach muscles flatten down and lengthen rather than bulking. The more the breathing is coordinated with the action, the harder this exercise.

Repeat 10–15 times.

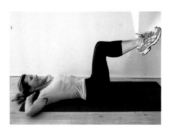 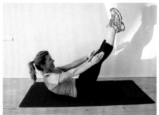 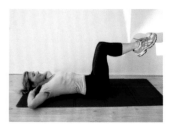

Stretch Sequence

1. Frog *Areas stretched: inner thigh.*

On a mat, sit down and hold the ankles towards you.

Stay for about 15 seconds or longer.

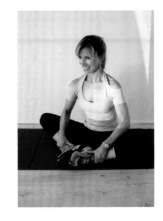

2. Forward Reach *Areas stretched: hamstrings, back of thigh.*

From a sitting position on the floor, extend one leg forward and ease the upper body towards the lengthened leg. To increase and broaden the stretch, turn the torso and opposite shoulder slightly more towards the straightened leg.

Hold for 15 seconds or longer and change sides.

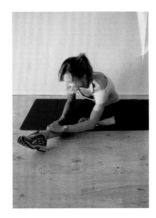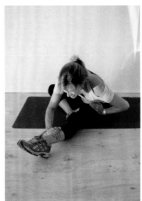

3. Glute Stretch *Areas stretched: buttocks.*

Lying on the back, with your right hand take the right knee towards the chest and direct it towards the left shoulder. Make sure the hips don't lift off the floor. Feel the stretch here for a few seconds before holding the right foot with the left hand and ease the foot towards you to increase the stretch. Make sure the knee is still directed towards the left shoulder.

Hold for 15 seconds or more and change sides.

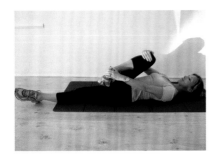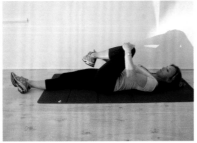

4. Variation of Glute Stretch *Areas stretched: inner thigh.*

Rest the right foot across the left bent knee. Wrap the arms around the left leg and pull it gently towards the chest.

Hold for 15 seconds or longer and change sides.

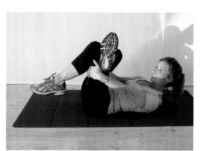 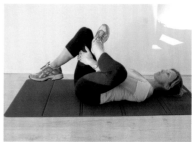

5. Splits in Second Position *Areas stretched: inner thigh.*

Lying on your back, ease both legs out to the side and add a little pressure to the split with the hands on the inner thigh.

Hold for 15 seconds or longer and slowly bring the legs up and back together.

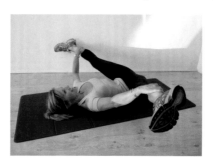

The Filler Workout

This workout is designed to go between the days of your weights workout. So that the muscles aren't overloaded and have time to repair, it is best to do your other chosen workout (either the Starter, Intermediate or Experienced) on alternate days or at least three times in the week. In between those days you may want to raise the metabolism much more to really give your body a chance to shape up and lose surplus fat. This is where the **Filler Workout** comes in.

All these workouts are planned around the heart rate going up and down, so that it peaks and recovers before going up again. This Filler Workout is short and explosive and will make sure that your body maintains a high metabolism for long beyond its duration.

These short, high intensity workouts are considered to keep the metabolic rate high for as long as 30 hours or more. Whereas the longer, steady, exercise sessions like jogging or aerobics, may only keep the metabolism elevated for 8 hours.

The emphasis of these following exercises is on raising the heart rate and taking very short rests between. Any suggested rest will be indicated.

1. Squats

Position the feet hip distance apart and bend from the hips and knees. Keep the knees in line with the toes and allow the arms to swing forward and back to warm up the shoulders.

Repeat 20–25 times.

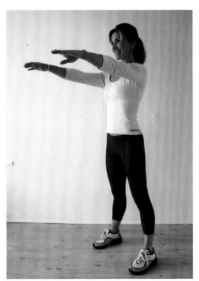 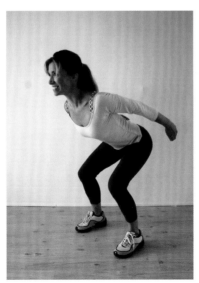 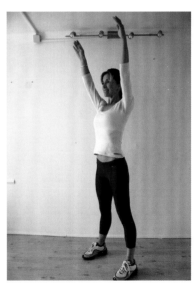

2. Heel Flicks

Bend both legs and transfer the weight to one foot while flicking the other foot towards the backside.

Repeat 16–20 times.

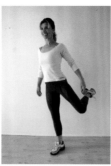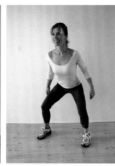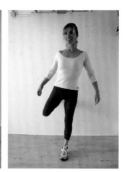

3. Bend and Side Reach

Continue with the bend and transfer of weight and reach over to one side and the other. Add a twist and rotation as you reach.

Repeat 10 times.

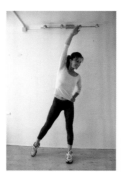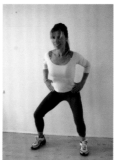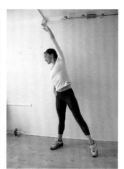

4 & 5. Knee Drives

Raise the knee high and lower behind while driving the arms in the opposite direction, as if running.

Repeat 8 each side.

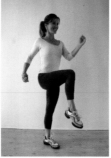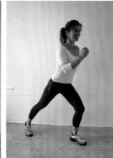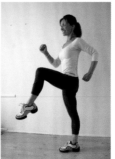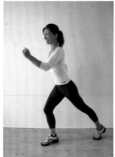

6. Swing Rounds

With both hands, hold each end of one weight. Push the weight out sideways at waist level, swing it round with the arms straight to the other side and pull it inwards. Push outwards from that side and swing straight to the other side.

Repeat 16 times.

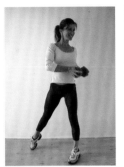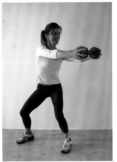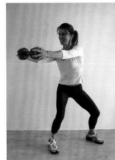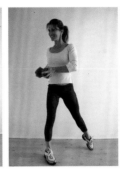

7. Step-ups

Using a stair, step ledge or something to step up on to, step up and down alternating legs.

Repeat 20 times.

PAUSE FOR 10 SECONDS

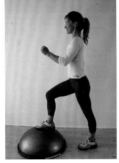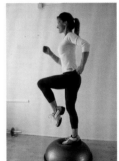

8 & 9. Wood Chops

Take the weight and hold it at each end. Lift the weight upwards and sideways and hold for a second before chopping it down diagonally to the other side while bending the knees and hold it here for a second, before swinging back up. Stay on the same side.

Repeat 10 each side.

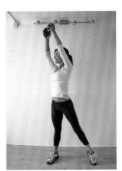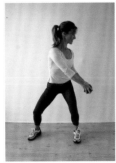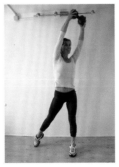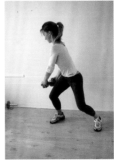

10 & 11. Sporty Feet

With the feet apart and weight mostly on the ball of the foot, stride across the other leg as if dashing about in a sport. Staying on the same side, bounce back and forth, keeping nice and agile while driving the arms with the action.

Repeat 10 each side.

PAUSE FOR 10 SECONDS

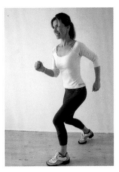 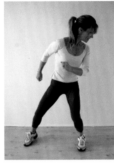 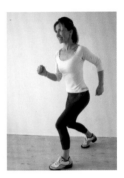

12 & 13. Swing Through

With one weight in a hand, and legs wider than hip distance apart, bend down with a straight spine and swing the weight through the legs. Keep the momentum and swing the weight back up high while straightening the legs. Keep the arm straight throughout. Stay on the same side for 8 repetitions.

Repeat 8 each side.

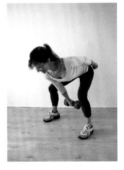 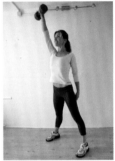

14. Split Jumps

With the left foot a stride further forward than the right, jump up and switch feet so that the right foot lands forward. Land in a light lunge.

Repeat 20 times.

PAUSE FOR 10 SECONDS

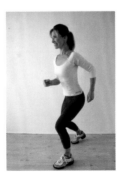 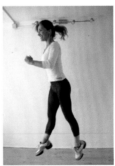 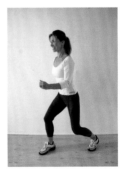

15. Floor Knee Raises

Place the hands and feet on the floor keeping the line between shoulders and heels straight. Separate the feet well to help with balance. Bring one knee towards the opposite hip then, as you place it back to its start position, bring the other knee in towards the opposite hip. Add a little bounce and speed to make it more intense.

Repeat 20 times.

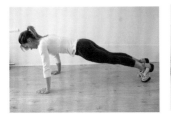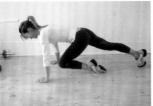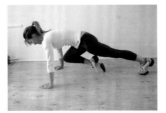

16. Turning Lunge Jumps with Step

Place one foot on the step, stair or ledge. Transfer the weight on to it and jump and turn while switching legs and land facing the other side. Make the jump high and the landing deep with a deep lunge on the outside leg.

Repeat 20 jump turns.

PAUSE FOR 10 SECONDS

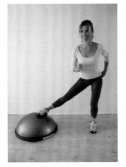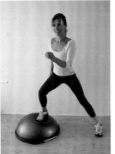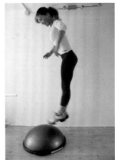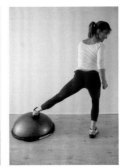

17. Jump-ups

Facing the step with the knees bent, jump up on to the step and land in a good squat bend. Step back down.

Repeat 15 times.

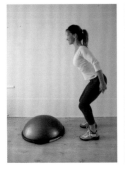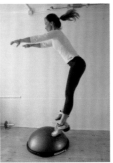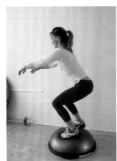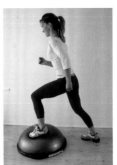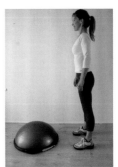

OUR LITTLE HABITS

Over time we get into routines and habits without even recognising them ourselves. It is only when you try to retrain yourself with new habits that you realise how habitual you have been over time.

For instance when you prepare meals, you might munch on a bit of this, snap off a bit of that, a handful of the other then a slurp of a drink. Then there might be a mid-morning snack of tea or a frothy coffee and biscuit, then a nice chunk of chocolate after lunch. It all adds up.

It isn't necessarily the extra calories that are the concern in this adding up. Don't think so much about the quantity of these treats and habits, but do consider the quality. This could all be extra toxins that your liver has to sort out just because of a few mindless actions!

How does insulin affect my fat and health?

Alongside the liver working overtime in a poorly balanced diet, the insulin-releasing pancreas will be too. Consider a hormone that makes you fat, ages you, increases your chances of heart disease and cancer, stresses you, raises the blood pressure and somewhere along the line creates diabetes. You'd want to control it wouldn't you?

Well that is insulin. Insulin is released rapidly after bad food choices. A bad food choice as you'll understand by now is one that converts to glucose rapidly during digestion. That means that your blood sugar levels will rise sharply which gives a burst of energy and, then, a bit of a slump. Then guess what? During that slump you'd fancy some more of that treat or, even think that you **need** some more of that type of food to 'get your energy levels up'.

You can see how this becomes addictive. In some respects there is little difference between drugs and fast foods; you get a high, then a low, then go looking for something else for a boost or quick pick-me-up. Both are pain numbing and we can start to understand why we fill our lives up with this junk. But were you aware that while we're fuelling up on food or habits as such, that the brain function goes into decline? It actually goes from operating as a conceptual being to basic reactions like that of a reptile: into 'fight or flight' mode!

Naturally, we have been trained, modelled and drilled to have better manners than that of a reptile but nonetheless, brain performance decreases and slight aggravation can send us into distorted thinking or unreasonable behaviour. This is especially evident among young children who haven't quite adopted manners yet. A bad diet leaves them with concentration problems, irritability, heightened emotions and socially it can be a struggle for all.

The knock-on effects of these little habits are, of course, vastly damaging. As the cycle continues, the adrenal production is on overload. Take a look again at the illnesses mentioned above to see what these two villains, insulin and adrenaline create.

REMEMBER

Watch out! The higher your consumption of food that turns to glucose quickly (refined foods, white pasta and bread, sugars etc.), the higher your insulin levels, as insulin is driven by glucose.

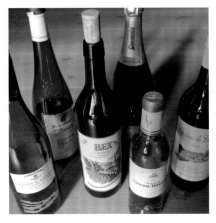

Based on one glass a day, six bottles of wine is what a 'light' drinker could get through in four weeks.

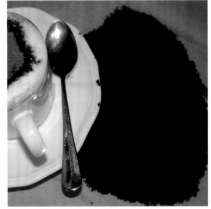

One coffee a day, which is a moderate consumption for some, adds up to looking like this much coffee over just one week

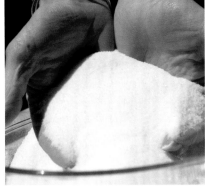

Cupped in these hands is 100 grams. This is easily consumed over a week. Imagine 4 times that amount passing through you over a month. This isn't even considering the occasional fizzy drink (see page 147).

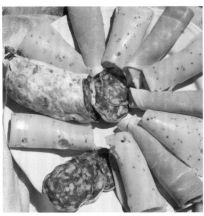

Processed food can go unrecognised and getting through a few packets of salami, ham or cheese is easily done over a few weeks.

REMEMBER

It is a good idea to have a visual understanding of how our habits add up. These photos are an example of what I show my groups at the end of our course.

A build up of modest consumption over four weeks could look like this.

Like an addict we keep fuelling the problem so health, mood, energy, output, concentration, sleep and emotions all take a hit from this. It is extremely wearing for the body. Not only that, while the blood sugar levels yo-yo like this, the body is storing fat. As that is what insulin allows the body to do – **store the fat**.

It would make sense therefore to understand the results of our little habits to our body. Does that treat or temptation outweigh the damage it does? Can you afford to feel tired or out of sorts later? And knowing how fluctuating blood sugar levels are a breeding ground for fat, do you still want to go ahead with that handful of habit?

With more knowledge of cause and effect, we can at least make informed decisions. Being aware is already a huge step forward. Reminding yourself to change habits is another step. Keeping to them most of the time is a huge stride towards great self-care and personal health care.

Looking at these pictures on page 135, think of how much during the 28 days of this plan, your liver won't have to deal with. These illustrate very modest habits, a glass of wine a day, one sugar in a daily hot drink. A pudding now and again and the hidden sugars in a seemingly healthy cereal and other sauces. And that is just 28 days.

Consider the amount over 6 months, a year, several years … with no break. It all adds up. And if losing fat is your desire, how about this for a calculation: 1 kilo of sugar is 3,600 calories, the equivalent of nearly two days eating for an average-sized, moderately active adult. It is about this many calories that makes ½ a kilo (1lb) of fat. In energy terms that would take about 10 hours of biking to shift! You can see how fat creeps on over time. And without this intake of sugar over a few months, the fat loss and improvement in health would be constant and impressive.

Knowing these figures, you can see how putting on a pound or kilo of fat takes some doing, when your weight on the scales fluctuates from morning to evening or from day to day, that can't be fat loss or fat gain but water changes. Fat comes on slowly, gram by unused gram and it leaves slowly. That is why, by getting the body into a healthy, natural balance, we can rely on it to mobilise surplus fat and toxins. This way, you can be sure that even if your weight on the scales isn't quick or dramatic to change, the workings within *are* changing for the better.

Another reason to follow the plan and food choices well, is that it will bump start, kick start, mobilise … however you want to phrase it … your body into using fat for its energy source. So when you come to fitting into clothes again, you can be sure this is fat loss, not water or muscle weight loss.

To lose 2 kilos of pure fat alone in one week is a big and unlikely deal unless the exercise programme is intensive. To lose 2 kilos in weight is more likely; a bit of fat and maybe a litre of water (equalling 1 kilo) will make up this weight loss. Sometimes there may be muscle loss too. This would be likely if the muscle isn't under enough demand or the individual isn't eating sufficiently. Since muscle is our energetic, fat-burning friend, we do all we can to keep it.

REMEMBER

If losing fat is your desire, how about this for a calculation: 1 kilo of sugar is 3,600 calories, the equivalent of nearly two days eating for an average-sized, moderately active adult.

It is about this many calories that makes ½ a kilo (1lb) of fat. In energy terms that would take about 10 hours of biking to shift!

More information **Visibly better health**

It isn't unusual that just after halfway through the plan, people admit to ailments that they used to have yet never thought them to be dietary, or 'little habit' related. But now that these spots, rashes, ailments or irritations have gone, why else would they have disappeared if it wasn't due to the cleaner and better eating habits?

Many are convinced their skin isn't as wrinkly or craggy as before starting the 28 day tidy up. And they are right. One of the most obvious things about someone having had a few weeks clear out is the colour in the skin, its plump texture and the luminosity. And if you don't notice it, others will.

An example of a body mass statistic reading

See how much more information this gives us than the scales. This person only lost 1 kilo on the scales but actually she had lost 3.5 kilo of pure fat, gained 1 kilo of muscle and was 1.5 litres more hydrated.

	Start of plan	End of plan
Total body weight	63 kilos	62 kilos
Muscle gain		1 kilo
Total body water	52 litres	53.5 litres (+1.5 kilos)
Body fat weight	22 kilos	18.5 kilos (-3.5 kilos)

When it comes to measuring body statistics at the end of the four week duration, there is always, a change for the better. For some reason we rely heavily on the scales to tell us the truth rather than how our clothes fit, how we look or the compliments that come from others. But the scales don't speak the truth in the case of health and fat loss.

Sometimes there may only be a loss of 1 kilo on the scales, but on further body composition measuring we see an improvement in hydration, say of 1.5 litres (1.5 kilos), plus a gain of up to a kilo of muscle therefore making a 2.5 kilo gain of body weight. So doing the maths correctly and according to the electric measuring device, that indicates a 3.5 kilo loss in pure fat. Remember the picture of fat on page 26? That was only 2 kilos. Imagine how much 3.5 kilos would look like.

Habits, as with weight fat gain, are insidious: gradual with a cumulative effect. Both creep up on you slowly, establish themselves well and then make themselves apparent in unsightly ways!

Since they probably started out as quite small in the beginning, if we are honest, habits don't tend to get better over time, just bigger. But we can of course take stock, knock these stalkers on the head and re-learn new and better ways.

So just visualise all those bad habits filtering through your liver over a four week period. You wouldn't give those baddies to your own pet so think before you consume them yourself. Then imagine how well the body could operate without having the strain of this amount for a few weeks. It would be like wasteland that got a break from being dumped on. There would be room for growth, new buds and blossoms.

Ditching bad habits for a while will allow energy, regeneration and renewal to flourish.

That is your inside dazzle making its way out. You can't buy that look, you can only cultivate it.

More information

There always comes a time midway through the 28 day course that I receive panic calls and questions from people. Their queries are normally along the lines of 'I lost 2 kilos in the first week and now it has stopped, what has happened?'

It takes a lot of reassurance to trust that the body is quietly doing its own thing in its own time and all we can do is support it, be patient and await the changes.

How can caffeine and some kinds of food make me fat?

That expression 'fight or flight', what does it mean in terms of the body and its reaction? Here's an explanation: to cope with a scary or dangerous situation, the body will release adrenalin. A rush of adrenalin will bring a surge of energy that will assist with either fighting or fleeing our way out of a threatening situation. It will fuel the areas of necessity for the task, like the heart, lungs and muscles. The body is prepared and focused for the matter it believes is at hand. All perfectly designed for a rocky encounter.

We can also stimulate the release of adrenalin with stimulants such as coffee, sugar, simple carbohydrates (bread, biscuits, cakes etc.), smoking and drinks containing caffeine. However, after having a piece of cake or a cigarette and with the adrenaline now surging, we don't get up and lay into someone or, charge off in a sprint for our life. We just sit there and feel the buzz.

This is when that extra release of energy is redundant. So instead it gets laid down as fat. Summed up: stress and stimulants disrupt insulin levels and therefore, over time, make you fat.

It is quite likely that most of the time you don't even feel the effects of these foods and their reaction to the body. That isn't because you are immune to them but because, rather like an addict, you don't feel the hit any more. Or you do feel it and actually believe you need that hit to operate throughout the day.

By now you will understand better as to why some foods just aren't digestive friendly. And that is what this plan is about. Putting good food inside you that will give the body a chance of peace. It is about getting it to operate from neutral again.

QUERIES AND QUESTIONS

What is so important about water and hydration?

Fluid is essential to this plan and everyday living. We can live without food for quite a while, but a lack of fluid is catastrophic. However getting fluid intake right is also important. For instance, a tired, dehydrated athlete after huge exertion has to be careful to re-hydrate slowly. The 'electrolyte' balance in this case is vital (see Day 5 of messages about electrolytes).

In fact it is best for all to drink throughout the day rather than vast amounts in a couple of sittings. As for the quantity of fluid, it is of course quite relative to an individual's size, exertion and climate that he or she lives in. I am small, but while racing through jungle day and night, I needed as much as 8 litres per day. At high altitude you dehydrate more without knowing as perspiration is quickly evaporated in higher and dryer air, airplanes likewise. So consider your activity and climate but as a general rule, 1.5 litres per day is adequate.

However you may come across information encouraging you to drink much more than this with the 'more the better' approach. Be wary of over doing the hydration side of things, cleansing as it may seem, too much water can flood the organs and impair their performance.

Bottled water is everywhere we go now and saves us from gastric upsets when travelling in areas with different sanitary systems from our own. But put under some rather interesting tests, it doesn't seem as spring fresh as we are led to imagine.

It is encouraging to hear that water in the UK actually exceeds the rigorous cleansing requirements and the tap water, up and down the country, out performs some bottled varieties, whilst costing an infinite amount less. The process of bottling water is costly in another area too; a single 1 litre bottle takes many litres of water to produce.

Dr Masaru Emoto pioneered work on water from an energetic perspective; the effects that vibration and consciousness has on water. Among many other studies and analysis, he has taken samples from lakes, rivers, reservoirs and taps from around the world, frozen them and then examined the micro clusters and crystals that formed. He discovered that water in its frozen state illustrates its true self.

While the conclusion that most city water doesn't compare to alpine springs is unsurprising, yet the difference in crystal formation from one source to another is extraordinary. Beautiful, symmetrical, delicate star or pentagon shaped crystals from free flowing, fresh sources of water, compared to clumpy irregular, darkened shapes from still and vitality-devoid water, makes a startling visual contrast.

Obviously tests were more extensive but another alarming fact is how water's energetic composition responds to ambiance. Playing certain styles of music from heavy metal to classical compositions, the crystals form exquisite or deformed shapes, depending on the vibration. It isn't exclusively classical music that creates the more beautiful crystal (and some classical music certainly didn't at all), modern and uplifting music has the same effect too in producing peaceful perfect crystals, whereas a sorry ballad has rather the opposite effect. Even crystal samples taken from a lake where there was a history of disturbance, distress and drowning, reflected trauma.

It is both inspiring and chilling to think that water responds to such variables other than pollution as we know it. It actually responds to attention and an intention. Far-fetched as that may seem, consider this a step further. Since our bodies are on average 60% fluid, imagine the influence that our intentions or moods, let alone incidents around us, have on us beyond the immediate emotional response.

In conclusion, water (including our own body) is best if it is kindly cared for! So gulped from the springs would be the best choice. Second to that, flowing from your tap. Laying still in bottles may mean it is sterile but it is not alive or flowing!

Since so much water is treated, distilled or filtered now, it is devoid of minerals. Prevent that kind of water from zapping more out of your body by getting into the habit of adding a pinch of sea salt to every litre.

How long after eating should I do the exercises?

Planning your exercise times is important so that you fit them in and so that they don't clash with a meal digesting. You may find that you can fit them in nicely first thing in the morning, before the house awakes or before chores begin. The advantage of this is that you are exercising on an empty stomach. So long as you do this reasonably soon after waking up you shouldn't suffer hunger or dizziness. On the other hand, afternoons and evening may suit you best. In which case allow 2 hours from your latest food before exercising and time your snack or meal for just after the workout.

More information **Allowing time for digestion**

Remember being told that you shouldn't go swimming straight after eating? That was right, not just for swimming, but for any activity.

The body is busy digesting after eating so not only will any activity or anxiety disrupt that digestion, the body can get cramp, and in the swimming pool, nobody wants that.

Digestion takes up a lot of energy. In fact it is believed it requires 50% of the body's energy to digest. It makes sense therefore not to place any kind of exertion on the body after eating.

That way, it can function well and ensure all the nutrients are absorbed. Rushing around after a meal will just inhibit the absorption and digestive process.

We often wonder how on a diet of red meats, wine and other foods we consider poor to our health, that the Mediterraneans have fewer health problems than the Northern Europeans!

Could it be something to do with siestas? That is a good amount of time to digest the food and reap the benefits of an hour or so of stress-free relaxation.

I find I'm going to the lavatory a lot.

In the first few days the body is busy shedding unwanted water that it has been holding while trying to buffer the cells' chemical imbalance. This will mean more visits to the lavatory and passing water. Don't slow down on your drinking and keep sipping water throughout the day. The body soon finds its balance, and visits to the loo will become less frequent!

What role does protein have in this plan?

Apart from having many essential nutritional benefits, protein is slow to be broken down in digestion and so therefore takes time to be converted to glucose. This means it helps with creating steady blood sugar levels. As mentioned in Day 3's message, protein also releases a chemical to the brain giving a signal of a satisfied appetite.

I thought that too much protein wasn't good for you.

Too much animal protein does not suit everybody and certainly a high consumption of cooked meat stresses the kidneys. Even vast quantities of nuts and seeds can be troublesome for the liver. But small quantities of many other things can also cause more problems. Keep a sensible balance in your meal portions and note that as little as 10% of protein on your plate will help with hunger, cravings and stabilising blood sugar levels. Protein from two-legged species tends to be preferable for digestion over cattle and red meat. Find the level of protein that suits you and keep it varied. Go to page 47 to select a broad protein choice of both vegetable and animal proteins and be assured that protein contains essential nutrients for the brain and body.

Apart from yogurt, there is no dairy produce in this plan. What about calcium?

We have been brought up to believe that dairy is the richest form of calcium. The problem is that so many are intolerant or at least sensitive to milk products. This may be because we pasteurise dairy produce. Even a cow's own calf would die if it was raised on pasteurised milk. It may also be that dairy is thought to cause more mucus which inhibits the absorption of nutrients. Read more about mucus on the next page.

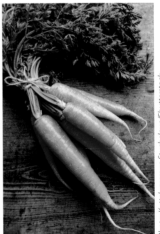

What is important is to consume calcium that your body will absorb well. As mentioned in Day 4's message, the body can assimilate with the calcium from carrots more easier than it can a glass of milk. Take a look at the other sources of calcium that are listed there.

Photo: Kuttelvaserova Stuchelova/Shutterstock

I've taken to eating lots of fish but I am now concerned about the levels of mercury I could be consuming.

Indeed this may be a consideration, but the mercury content of a fish due to its habitat is minimal. If you've ever had mercury fillings in your teeth or vaccinations, the quantity of mercury in these would far outweigh that of a fish, and could be much more of a concern.

I usually take vitamin tablets as supplements to my diet. Will I get sufficient nutrients if I stop them during the detox?

Nature gave us a variety of foods that support, heal and nourish the body. The body knows how to digest and absorb this food, it also knows how to reject their overload. Tablets have no live enzymes, do not assimilate with the body and can therefore not be in harmony with digestion. We speak in milligrams of vitamins required, but the body will select its needs from wholesome food and eliminate at its limit. Supplements are not a natural form, the body does not recognise them and can therefore not measure or metabolise the overload. Tests after consumption of supplements may well show improved levels in the blood, but the body's complexity is infinite. Respect its delicate chemical balance and fuel it with fresh choices.

What about organic versus other produce?

Tests have been run on this subject but their conclusion was not of much value to us as consumers. There's no doubt that the chemicals on non-organic produce do us no favours and may cause havoc to our health and environment, but as to whether their nutrient composition is compromised, it isn't believed so. Although there are other reports which claim that produce grown in a natural, non-pesticide environment, has to naturally produce more antioxidants in order to survive.

More information **Mucoid plaque**

Some are of the belief that dairy (with the assistance of processed food) creates 'mucoid plaque'. Some admit to dairy increasing mucus levels but this substance is a different level. Mucoid plaque is said to be a vile smelling, rubbery lining that sticks to the intestines and makes a breeding ground for less than perfect health.

After hearing about this toilet phenomenon, this stuff had to be expelled and Emiko and I bought a kit. This kit was a mix of herbs and a digestive absorber.

At first it seemed very efficient, the bowels emptied out and felt much lighter and by the second day there was significant evidence of the mucoid plaque, near enough a metre in length.

Then we became suspicious. Each portion of powder and juice brought on a swollen belly followed by more of this new age cleanse. If the large intestines are not even 2 metres long, how long can this purge continue for?

Were the ingredients in the kit creating the very condition we were trying to eradicate?

Unattractive as it was, it wasn't vile smelling and, on better inspection of the substance purged, it appeared to be a clay-like binding substance. We ran a home made test with the kit in water; within two hours, a slimy gloop formed which, with a bit of digestive acid and bowel action, would have been the exact resemblance of the snake-like mucoid plaque we were trying to expel. Further research lead us to the understanding that, as with many things, some kits were more pure and better than others. But additionally and probably more poignant, neither gastroenterologists in endoscopies or pathologists during autopsies encounter this condition.

However, the clean and converted swear by it. Quite rightly, they say that until you've expelled the vile substance you can't claim it doesn't exist. Maybe a different kit is in order …

For the purpose of *Tidy the Temple* and keeping a toxic-free body, choose organic where it is feasible for you. There are plenty of reasons to opt for organic and a better taste is one of them. Remember too, beyond *Tidy the Temple*, that anything edible that has grown in plant form, despite its environment, will still be superior to any manmade alternative.

Why during the first stage of the plan, do I get spots and other symptoms of toxicity when normally, I never get these ailments?

When we are happily eating our packet, refined or less than fresh food, the body goes into emergency mode to rebalance the contamination. This means that the white blood cells flock to the place of trouble, in this case, the digestion. Their work is full time trying to solve the toxic overload.

When we remove the problem of contamination there is no point of emergency and the body has time and energy to literally purge poisons. This purge may come in different ways for different people, such as headaches, spots, rashes, sore joints, night sweats etc. This is why it is so essential to let the body go through this process thoroughly without the interruption or disturbance caused by chemicals, pain killers and other unnatural sources.

I'm a sufferer of inflammation in my joints and I felt really quite unwell during the first stage of the plan.

It isn't unusual that this type of complaint has an extreme reaction during the tidying up plan. Removing sugar and caffeine from the diet can have some extraordinary results. Some talk of not just joint ache but a fever for a day or so. Yet following the discomfort comes relief of pain and 'having not felt so good in ages'. Contrary to common belief, a temperature is the body's way of healing and killing off unwelcome bacteria. Be brave, trust your body and let it work through the phase on its own!

Is salt good or bad?

Salt has had a lot of bad press over the years and whether we should eliminate salt during a *Tidy the Temple* course is a frequently asked question.

Associations with high blood pressure and inflexible arteries are some of the links made between salt and an assault on our health. But the impact that salt has alone is marginal compared to other lifestyle choices that encourage such conditions. As with many food types, there are good and poor quality, along with refined and non-refined options to choose from. For instance it is the refining process in table salt that adds chemical toxins and strips it of the magnesium mineral content. Table salt is certainly to be avoided.

Whereas unrefined salt is something the body benefits from. In its original state it is packed with minerals that are essential for good health; good cell pH and electrolyte balance, regulating blood sugar and bone development to name a few.

It is this high content of sodium that has been the concern for elevating blood pressure. Yet left in its natural state, the magnesium content offsets the sodium balance.

As with everything in nature, it is balanced and whole, serving a purpose within a chain of sequences. It is mostly man's changes that disrupt that equilibrium. So keeping salt in its natural state means we can enjoy the extra flavour it brings to dishes.

When following *Tidy the Temple*, we can be in control of the salt quality that we're using but beyond the plan there is less chance. Since salt is added to many things from toothpaste to cereal, it becomes a component in so much that we consume – and it's unlikely to be the better variety. This means the addition of salt to your diet is not the starting point of salt consumption, but rather the layering on to the 'hidden' salt that you are consuming elsewhere.

Are soy products healthy?

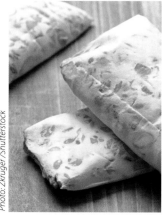

Photo: Zkruger /Shutterstock

Soya, tempeh and tofu are all from the same family, the soybean. The soybean is classed as a legume but is more of an oilseed than a pulse. It is rich in protein and so considered an excellent vegetarian alternative to animal protein. Whereas tofu is made from the curd of soy milk, tempeh is higher in protein as it uses the whole soybean. It is also richer in taste than tofu.

While soy has been used for thousands of years in the East, it has only grown in popularity relatively recently in the West since World War II. Now America and Brazil are its biggest producers and the profits are huge. Soy can be found in processed foods, oils, supplements, animal feed, pre-packed meals, dairy alternatives such as yogurt, cheese, ice cream and baby formulas, among many other products.

There are plenty of positive claims about soy, yet the evidence of direct health benefits is inconclusive. Although analysis shows that soy contains such minerals as calcium, magnesium and zinc, the body cannot assimilate the nutrients due to a high content of phytate (the principal phosphorus store in plants) in soy, which inhibits absorption of the minerals.

There is growing awareness that the plant based estrogens contained in soy products can encourage hormone abnormalities. For instance, a cup of soya milk can depress thyroid function for up to seven days. Since good thyroid function is integral to our health, energy, moods and many more vital bodily interactions, it is advisable to keep any thyroid upset or interruption to a minimum.

Phytate can normally be reduced through long, slow cooking processes, yet the phytate found in soy is resistant. However, a successful technique for reducing the phytate content is by a long period of fermentation. This makes the nutrients easily assimilated. Tempeh and soy sauce are therefore the preferred options from the soybean. Keep the other unfermented products to a minimum.

MOVING ON FROM HERE

You've completed your four week clean out, seen and felt how good the changes are so, now what?

To fall back into old habits straight away would actually be harder than you think. Firstly your body will be only too quick to object and show you symptoms of disapproval – those same symptoms that you lived with before *Tidy the Temple* but maybe did not consider to be so diet related.

Does that mean the body is more sensitive than before? No, it is just operating from a better place and you are more in tune with what works for you and what doesn't. This is good, and it could mean that you won't blindly step into a state of disease over time. It also means that you'll understand the reason for a headache, throat irritations, spots, gas, feeling irritable etc. and steer yourself away from the cause. Of course I am well aware from my own deep experiences that diet and self-care don't fix everything. But it does support the body and mind and so can reposition you for the best chances of moving forward.

Once you have completed the 28 days of tidying your temple, you'll have a much clearer feeling of what foods work for you and how much command they have on how you look and feel.

Take a look at the **Moving Forward** section of the recipes for great dishes that satisfy taste and tummy yet still sit the right side of good self-care.

Keeping to even a few of these *Tidy the Temple* points beyond the 28 days makes a difference. Habits are accumulative and over time, create change. Be honest enough to compare your new ways with your original ones and congratulate yourself, you glow from the inside out now.

There may be the odd celebration or outing that throws the rhythm that you've worked so hard to create, but just let it go. Life is about going with the tide and then navigating to the best choice. Just get back into the habits that serve your health best, whenever you can.

It is important though, with any food or drink that you haven't had for the duration, to bring them in as if feeding a baby, bit by bit. A big binge of sugar or alcohol, even normal things like bread, will leave you feeling unwell and the joy of the forbidden fruit is quickly tainted.

Not only will it leave you feeling rotten having had a binge, it does make the next day difficult. Coupled with cravings, tiredness and feeling under par, you will be inevitably reaching for poor choices. It is on days like this that discipline has to absolutely override fancies and feelings if you want to keep within the moderation rule.

The 80% good and 20% fun ratio is well known. 'Good' will mean different things to different people, as will 'fun'. I'm forever calculating how many 'fun' meals or snacks would make up to 20% per week but it never works out as straightforward as that.

Has my body become more sensitive to certain foods after this tidy up?

The body hasn't become more sensitive to these foods. It is simply that you will be in better tune with your body and so will be able to pinpoint reactions, and the cause of them.

Your body probably didn't tolerate toxic food or drink beforehand, but the symptoms of intolerance were most likely being masked by other conditions. Now it will be more evident which foods make you sleepy, bloated or anxious.

Symptoms to sensitivity and intolerance tend to be quite instant and apparent while the body is 'clean'.

Since there is no obvious monitor other than our knowledge and conscience, just keep an eye on each plate's balance. Is it more fun than healthy? Is there any raw food? How is the acid and alkaline balance? This isn't to suggest that you reject or refuse plates by any means, but it is to recommend that you develop your own 'eating-ometer' so that you can balance things out later on that day or week and, keep on top of feeling good, effortlessly.

Everyone that I've ever seen through this 28 day course manages to maintain the greater part of their new eating and exercise habits for some time beyond the course duration. This has a lot to do with giving the mind and body enough time to truly settle into the new fuel and new you. You get to a point when you don't want to sabotage feeling good.

During these weeks people learn the importance of snacking and keeping the blood sugar levels steady. But everyone takes away something different for what works for them. Interestingly even when I meet up with them a year on, they may say something along the lines of how they're 'not eating so well' or have 'got out of shape again'. Yet looking at them they look better than ever. Then they will admit to keeping to the skeleton of the plan and how much it has changed their understanding and perception of food. When I measure their body statistics again, they are closer to their best reading and measurements than they realised, and a long way off their initial out of shape readings. Often people forget how far they have come and think of any 'slip up' as not very good at all.

Anyone with high standards will recognise that trait of not seeing how far and well you have come, but how far you have to go. Admit it, you have done well, you've tidied up, you have straightened up your act. Now if some of that carries on for a while yet, that is huge progress.

A whole 28 days of renewal has been allowed without interruption. If this was repeated every 12 months, think of the rejuvenation and glow that you'd be allowing yourself over time. Instead of ageing and feeling like your years have caught up with you, you'd be holding back the clock on degeneration. Add the weeks into months and months into years, and you'll appreciate the significant upgrade that you will have made to your vitality.

As mentioned earlier, it is believed that it takes between 21 and 28 days to change habits. This is one of the reasons why staying tight to the programme during our duration together was important. As anyone knows, the odd 'slip up' makes it harder for the next few days to get back on the wagon. Then, that willpower is required as the inclination to choose healthy options gets a little corrupted. However, the best way to see this is that you have given your body a rest from toxins for 4 weeks. Thanks to eliminating our bad habits that inhibit rejuvenation and cell repair, the body has been able to settle into regenerating at a good pace.

You have found a way that works for you and to keep many of these new habits would of course bring further improvements. When you think how long we can slowly spend getting ourselves into a toxic state, it would be great to balance that somehow, with healthier habits.

Gaining the lost fat again

If we had been on a calorie-reduced diet, yes, it would be quite likely that you would gain all the lost fat quickly again. Someone who has been to diet club may keep going back to diet club. That is because diets that reduce calories change the Fat Set Point. This is the hormone that dictates your metabolism. So these people cut down their food, get hungry, their metabolism slows down to accommodate the lack of fuel and, as soon as the regime is over, the fat is easily stored again due to a sluggish metabolism. During *Tidy the Temple*, you did it differently. You possibly ate more than before, and you ate regularly. This keeps the metabolism working, not to mention putting demand on the muscle fibres as you have with the exercise sessions. If you're feeling like you've piled on the weight, it is likely that it is mostly water retention.

Consider that 3,500 calories (thereabouts) is equivalent to ½ a kilo of fat. So to gain 1 kilo of pure fat takes some doing. To gain a kilo of weight, as you will know, is easier. Now that you know how to keep your body in a good pH balance you will naturally have less bloating and this allows the body to operate from a point of balance, and therefore mobilise fat more easily.

So, in short, there is no need to obsess or think your good work will be quickly undone. I really do encourage you to follow these practical points where possible:

Starch and carbohydrates

Eating carbohydrates regularly can squeeze out the space for more important nutrients found in salad and vegetables. I'm not advocating the 'no carbs' rule at all. Just don't let them overrule proportionally on your plate, or at least try the rotation suggestion mentioned in Day 11: one day on, the next day off. This will keep from falling into that 'feeling sluggish' trap and wanting more starch 'to give you a kick'. The same goes for the REFINED food and flour-based foods. A little less of these types of foods will make a big difference to your health and condition over the weeks, months not to mention a year.

Breads and flours

As mentioned in Day 11, there are a variety of flours such as rye, corn, spelt, buckwheat, rice and quinoa. These make good baking options and they tend not to cause the digestive aggravation that wheat without slow-acting yeast can.

Watch out for the sugar

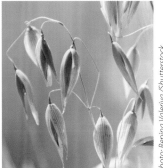

Photo: Repina Valeriya /Shutterstock

Sugar creeps into diets quietly. It starts with sweeter and exotic fruits, then gets extended to honey or other natural sweet sources and before you know it, not a day goes past without sugar. It sneaks in and throws insulin levels and therefore your mindset. If we are to have a pudding or pastry four times a week, a teaspoon of sugar in a cup of tea per day, the odd bowl of cereal, a little sauce here and there, that would add up to about a kilo of sugar.

Make sure your sugar intake (if you really want it) is controlled by you, with choices like raw cane sugar, molasses and honey as sweeteners. These all have their nutrient qualities and, in small doses, offer something. But they still set the blood sugar levels off. The refined white sugar should go. You'll find enough of it outside home and hidden in hams, jams, cereals and juices etc. Keep to the pure, original state stuff and only now and again.

Sugar variations

Molasses as a syrup or in granules Molasses contains small amounts of calcium, copper, iron and is rich in potassium.

Pure raw cane sugar This has similar qualities to molasses.

Honey (ideally from your region). Depending on the quality it is anti-bacterial and anti-fungal.

Stevia Another natural sweetener to consider is Stevia. Stevia is a small easy growing shrub originally from South America where it has enjoyed enormous popularity for years. Now the rest of the world has woken up to it and its usage is spreading globally.

Due to the density of its taste, Stevia is best used as a sweetener rather than for baking where volume and weight help perfect the pudding! For instance where you would use a cup of raw sugar, you would only need two teaspoons of Stevia. A teaspoon of sugar will equate to an eighth of a teaspoon of Stevia.

There is a slightly bitter aftertaste but most importantly, here is a natural sweetener that doesn't affect blood sugar or insulin levels nor does it encourage cravings like many other sugar based food. Ensure you buy a good quality stevia for both taste and health benefits.

Remember, sugar, no matter its form, still converts to glucose quickly and will set the blood sugar levels off on a roller coaster.

Artificial sweeteners

Hopefully after all you have learnt and practised during your tidy up, anything artificial won't feature on your shopping list. But out of curiosity you may wonder if they have the same effect as sugar on the insulin/blood sugar levels. No, they don't. But they will open up your appetite for sweeter foods. Don't invite them into your Temple!

Keep going with the snacks

These will keep blood sugar levels steady which is key to health and making good food choices. Just watch that these snacks stay clean and simple: fruit or veg and a hint of protein. An apple on its own won't do the job. If you're regularly reaching out for bread and cheese as a snack, think of some better choices. Also bear in mind the acid and alkaline options.

If you go out for a meal

Before you go out for a meal, have a small snack an hour or so before. Fruit and nuts or vegetables and a light protein would be good. Keeping the blood sugar

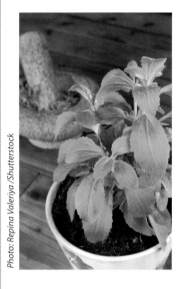

Photo: Repina Valeriya /Shutterstock

levels steady means you won't approach the meal out with too much gusto. It also means you will choose according to your needs rather than because you're feeling famished. And, you won't eat all the bread while waiting for your meal!

Acid and alkaline

Be mindful to have a balance of this in each meal. This keeps the cells happy more than anything. Keep reducing the quantity of acidic foods making sure you have alkaline foods to bulk up with. We need both, in balance. If you find that you have a heavily acidic balanced day, get juicing and juice mostly vegetables. Refer to the list of Acidic and Alkaline foods on page 90 for a reminder.

Dairy

Many believe that dairy is rich in calcium and I still come across articles in health magazines supporting it. But, unless it is unpasteurised, the body doesn't assimilate dairy products, so how can it absorb the nutrients? Most people say they feel better without dairy. Another option is to try goat's and sheep's yoghurt, which is easier on digestion. In any case keep dairy in moderation and be sure to get calcium through other foods listed in Day 4's message, page 60.

Vitamins and supplements

I used to take loads and spend a heap of money on them. Now I wouldn't. But I leave that with you and your own thoughts or experiences. In affluent countries there is no famine and plenty of honest food available. Nature brings us leafy greens for calcium, carrots for vitamin A, citrus fruit for ascorbic acid and an abundance of nutrients from other plants. How can anything substitute that?

Vitamins are, of course, important, but in the correct and most natural measure. Read more about supplements in the Queries section. Keep the vitality in the food you consume. Overcooking devitalises and demineralises, so cook or steam lightly and opt for raw produce when possible. A juicing machine is a great way forward. It is easy on the digestive system, packed with nutrients and live enzymes and great for getting vitamins in when you feel something lurking. Also, a fresh juice is an easy way to get vitamins into children. Read Day 25 for more about juicing.

Oils

You will see in the recipe sections how nut oils replace butter for cooking. Unrefined oils are costly but oils that are refined, hydrogenated and highly heated are damaging to our health long-term. Most oils' structure is altered for the worse when cooked at high temperatures. If unrefined oils don't fit your budget, coconut oil is excellent; it comes solid, it is tasteless and doesn't change its composition if heated at temperatures lower than 170 degrees. It also makes a great body moisturiser. Just make sure it is a non-hydrogenated coconut oil.

Essential fatty acids

The human brain is made up of fatty acids, yet the body cannot produce its own fatty acids. Therefore it is critical that our diet makes significant provision for them, hence the name Essential Fatty Acids (EFAs) or Omegas as you may also know them.

If you want to lift your moods, improve concentration, reduce cravings, increase your energy levels, get fitter and stronger, improve recovery, have beautiful skin, tan more and burn less in the sun, then a daily dose of Essential Fatty Acids is what you need.

And the positives don't stop there. This fabulous fat also promotes our natural steroid production meaning we can upgrade our athletic performance effectively and naturally. It also acts as a natural protector to our bodies from toxins and pollutants. When food rich in EFAs was given to juvenile delinquents under test conditions, they became more responsive in a positive way.

Their benefits are vital. We can find a good balance of EFAs in avocados and some greens but especially in oils such as flaxseed, hemp, coconut, sunflower seed and wheatgerm.

Here's to mostly good and healthy choices and a bit of fun food now and again!

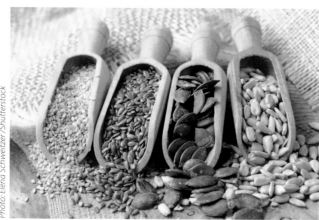

Photo: Elena Schweitzer /Shutterstock

PREGNANCY, PARENTING AND PERSONALLY SPEAKING

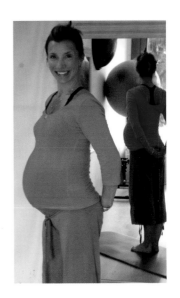

I couldn't help but notice that after each *Tidy the Temple* course I ran, there were a number of pregnancies! Each course would attract about 30 or more ladies, and often two or more would fall pregnant immediately afterwards. Once there were five, myself included. And three of the five were 40 plus years old. Emiko became pregnant with Arthur, shortly after another course that I ran. I don't believe that any of us were really 'trying' for a baby but we felt lucky all the same.

This isn't to claim that *Tidy the Temple* is a guaranteed fertility booster but equally, healthy habits do change the expression of the body. Eating well and exercising moderately can only set you up for the better.

Every pregnancy is different, even if the mother's habits seem to be the same. Energy levels and vulnerabilities to conditions can vary and what worked for the previous pregnancy, may well not respond the same for the following.

The baby takes all it needs from mum so it is easy for mum to feel depleted and lacking all of a sudden. Blood pressure, blood count, iron levels and sugar levels can all turn one way or another and that's without mentioning other irritants and aches that a tough pregnancy may present.

Thinking ahead

Eating foods from the fields rather than the factories is going to at least help, if not overcome all the ailments associated with pregnancy. Fighting hunger and cravings with packaged meals and fluffy breads will only impact on your energy and spark and provide more fat to shift post birth.

Maintaining healthy habits whilst pregnant makes returning to good health and shape after giving birth a much easier task. Once baby arrives, there is much less time for you and any hopes of regular scheduled exercise can go out of the window! So being a little ahead of the game and staying there throughout pregnancy will pay off. Disturbed nights and less sleep are also likely to be a factor which can further deplete energy and dampen any inclination to focus on a weight loss and toning up plan.

Finding the balance

During my pregnancies I followed the latter stages of the *Tidy the Temple* plan. The complex carbohydrates such as barley and rice now and again, felt satisfying and right. With those options there is normally no bloating or digestive aggravations to our insides that are becoming more compacted as a foetus grows. The regular consumption of protein with all meals and snacks helps keep the extra quota required while pregnant. Choose organic options where possible and keep expanding with the vegetarian proteins.

Any cravings were under control although I still enjoyed a few baked delights from the **Moving Forward** recipe section! My latest pregnancy was such a celebration

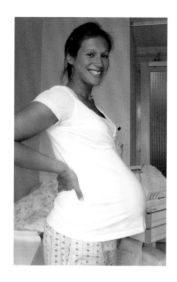

that I rejoiced in feasting on Emiko's puddings sometimes. Having been harder on myself with more restrictions in the previous pregnancy and the outcome being so tragic, there was an element of understanding that you can do things to apparent perfection and still not be in control of the results.

My principle was for regular and light eating, a good balance of acid and alkaline along with plentiful portions of raw and fresh food that the body could understand, digest and assimilate. There wasn't much more to do without creating unnecessary pressure.

Essential

Omega 3, 6 and 9 become especially important during pregnancy. These are essential fatty acids which keep the brain in balance. Without them there is reduced learning, more anxiety and diminished ability to feel happy. Though the brain is largely composed of fatty acids, the body can't make these fats, hence the usage of *essential*. These fats are the baby's principal nourishment via the placenta and the demand increases in the latter weeks so mum's reserve decreases. The depletion continues with breast feeding so if her reserves are already low, she will become further lowered and can descend into depression or the 'baby blues' as they are known. Get enough omega 3, 6 and 9 from oily fish, flaxseed, sesame seed, hempseed (or their oils) and coconut oil.

The benefits of essential fatty acids are broad and eye opening. Go to the 'Moving on from here' section to find out more about them in *'Oils'*.

Iron

Now and again pregnant ladies become iron deficient or anaemic. In my pregnancies, I encountered nurses all too keen to give a shot of iron to increase levels and bolster blood test results. Even if it is showing a higher reading in the next blood test, it doesn't mean the body itself has absorbed it as if from natural source and via ingestion. A vastly experienced naturopath with success stories in turning health around, even declares iron injections to be toxic to the body.

So how do we find iron? Iron supplements are one of the best sellers, but let's look into how we can find it naturally and therefore benefit wholly from it. Women need more than men, and pregnant women need all the more. Dark-leafed vegetables and salad will bring a percentage of your iron needs, so where you can't eat enough of them, push them through the juicer. Two cups of raw spinach will offer nearly half of your needs and added to your morning omelette, there's only need for a few more iron rich options. Pumpkin seeds are a good example and three tablespoons alone, scattered into fruit salads, salads or grains, will bring about a quarter of your requirements. Dates make a nice sweet treat and around five of them can help you top up iron intake. A tablespoon of blackstrap molasses will soon have your iron levels reading well at any blood test!

Stress

Perhaps easier said than done, but stress is incredibly corrosive and should be kept to a minimum at any time, particularly during pregnancy. Limiting stress is important for baby's growth development and mother's health. Of course, babies are born in hideous and stressful environments all around the world all the time, but given the choice, seek peace over stress where possible.

Pregnancy can compound existing stresses, whether that be financial or the need for more practical and physical help. So support is crucial to the calming process.

Stress makes our body release cortisol and adrenaline into the bloodstream and excessive levels are to be avoided. This sunk in for me when being monitored for my most recent baby. Because of an oversight with the previous pregnancy, I was under regular and tedious testings. Measuring the baby's heart rate for 40 minutes at a time was one of the frequent observations. I got to know the baby's basic rhythm and beats per minute very well. It was between 118 and 130 depending on her activity in the womb.

One morning I attended yet another check up having not slept well after a night of turmoil. I forget the drama of the incident but I remember my husband and I being at loggerheads over something that was vital to me and of no significance to him. There were a lot of tears shed on my part.

Once my belly was strapped up with monitors again that morning, I was more than troubled to see that the baby's heart rate was now between 150 and 160 bpm, 12 hours after the disagreement. While I'd have hoped the stress hormones had passed through, it was a shock to see that the impact of the night was still meandering through our joined blood supply. Meanwhile the nurse was filling in my medical questionnaire,

'Any allergies Madame?'

'Yes, my husband.'

Endorphins

These hormones have an incredible tranquilising effect and their potency is far more powerful than morphine. Furthermore, we can double that shot by exercising. It takes as little as 15 minutes of exercise to activate endorphins and the effect can last for a few hours.

Getting out daily for a brisk walk or another form of invigorating exercise will help with endorphin release but, if your pregnancy is a tiring one and the thought of marching out daily doesn't appeal, be encouraged that just three times a week will still keep your happy hormones topped up.

Sunshine

While campaigns to avoid skin cancer urge us to stay out of the sun, the downside of not getting enough sun gets overlooked and creates deficiencies in itself. Apart from being a great mood lifter, it is also vital for vitamin D and therefore essential for baby's bone density and growth.

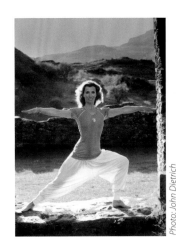

Photo: John Dietrich

Will I get my figure back?

Making *Tidy the Temple* an ongoing lifestyle has always meant great post pregnancy shape up because minimising digestive and absorption challenges means the body isn't battling too hard. After my pregnancies there was never many kilos of weight gain and even that was gone after a month. That doesn't mean I looked in shape but there weren't kilos of fat to deal with and firmness and body composition were always turned around within a couple of months.

Despite needing the six week or more recovery from C-sections, I was usually back into reasonable shape after three months. It was the same for Emiko and others who followed *Tidy the Temple* principles.

I was able to film DVDs, run courses and not need to make excuses or cover my tummy. This isn't to brag, but to illustrate that the *quality* of food is vital to regaining your figure. I have a big appetite and I do not go hungry, but I do pay attention to the balance of foods. This isn't a case of being lucky and naturally pinging back into shape but an example of giving the body assistance instead of hurdles.

The **scraggy skin** on mummy's tummy is a question I am often asked about. On many mothers I have seen this greatly improve and often disappear, even in the short period of the 28 day plan. When you see that skin, so slack and wrinkly, it is hard to believe it could reverse. But it can.

In Day 14 of the daily messages I mentioned regeneration and how many days and weeks parts of the body took to renew themselves. If the atoms within the cells are constantly changing, seize the opportunity to make today's actions, tomorrow's step towards better health. According to these ever flowing changes, your skin can be renewed within three weeks. That is, it can be the same old saggy state or firmer and more luminous.

The skin is our largest organ and a mirror of our health. Given the best opportunity for vitality it can be restored and rejuvenated, mummy tummy included. Having had three babies between the age of 38 and 45, I am no spring chicken for reproduction and can speak from personal experience. So can you expect skin to bounce back to youthful elasticity after pregnancy, like that of a 30 year old? **Yes** you can, despite age.

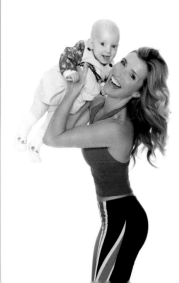

The body moves at its own pace and the best we can do is encourage and assist, rather than hinder and obstruct. Even after 9 months of changes, of growing and stretching, one month can make a considerable change for the better. At the same time, it would be wrong to say that these changes are for the long-term *if* good habits are not maintained. Mummy's scraggy tummy can make a comeback if neglected for too long. Nonetheless, it is encouraging to know the choice for better or worse is up to us.

Genetics will always play a role in body and health and it would be foolish to dismiss that. But many practitioners agree that genes are not deterministic and that 98% of the population can turn them off. 'Gene expression' is a term that is becoming more common. Simply put, this is how our genes communicate with our cells. Apparently we can actually change our relationship with our genes! Even with recurring conditions in generations, the individual needs to fuel and fire the inherited condition to activate it. The big question is how not to. Yet it doesn't take a genius to guess how we can modify the damage of rampant and insidious poisons. Just knowing we have a big say in our health and regeneration, is something that could feed our subconscious for the positive.

Personally …

No one in my family line found having babies as difficult as I did. I rather relied on that record and, coupled with my background in fitness, I thought there would be no troubles. How life teaches us! My first child involved a three day labour, many changes of staff shifts and a county council that wasn't keen for Caesarean budgets. 'Her lower section is going to burst,' I heard a midwife exclaim. It didn't that time, but an overdue C-section meant it was vulnerable second time round.

It didn't matter then and I had a beautiful baby boy. For the family's financial flow I needed to get the show back on the road as soon as possible. Within 6 weeks, I was demonstrating exercises at a fitness show at the NEC in Birmingham, another show in London, filming workouts for products or shopping channels and dragging dear baby Oscar around to keep him breast fed. He was breast fed until he began clamping his newly grown teeth at 10 months old. It was a busy first year that included relocating to a new country amongst other things. Then, just as my second pregnancy came, my father's health deteriorated.

I dropped work and responsibilities and returned for hospital visits. This was the man who'd skied to the Arctic, mountaineered in the Himalayas, started ballet at 67 years old, kept his men in work through two recessions. He'd taught me to shoot, dive, canoe, climb, forgive and battle on. But while others came and went in intensive care, my father stayed. I was four months pregnant so had just announced our news, then the bleeding started and the miscarriage begun. I lay in a hospital bed waiting for the baby to pass. At least, I thought, with this soul departing, my father's would stay.

My father died the next day. The baby would have been due around his birthday. It isn't that I expect life to be fair or without its tragedies but this one hit me flat. Losing my father had been a lifetime fear. Every expedition he went on I worried would be his last. The desolation of life without him lived up to my expectations. Apart from the obvious and excruciating void, it was also a slap in the face of how little control we have on life and losses and how misfortune is not rationed or spread evenly. Work and home life was a struggle.

My father, despite his faults, had been an unchallenged role model and with him now gone, other men seemed to pale by comparison – a common problem for a daughter, and no doubt their husbands! My husband is a musician and all that sensitivity and talent I'd once been allured by, now just resembled artistic temperament. I understood why in the old days, composers didn't live under the same roof as their families! If the ambiance at home was to be described in music, it'd have been modern jazz – exciting with some alarming discords.

Another pregnancy ensued immediately after running a *Tidy the Temple* course. With my history in mind and not my supposed genetics, I went to all extremes to make this a smooth labour. Many a relaxation, yoga move and mind over matter technique was exercised alone, and with therapists. I'd actually come to believe that a Caesarean was for those who got childbirth wrong! I was ready for this labour despite a pregnancy consumed by fatigue and ailments.

The labour was far from what I had rehearsed for. My womb burst, the baby died and an emergency Caesarean ensued. All those techniques I'd practised to making this a blissful moment were reduced to fanciful rubbish. My notes and cautions from the previous birth such as, 'avoid long labour, lower segment is weak … allergic reaction to Oxytocin', were more than ignored, they were performed. After the previous labour, 25 hours was nothing. But 25 hours of trauma, vomiting and rupturing from not being heard, made it a torturous mental and physical bloodbath.

However all that mental preparation had helped. Not in any way that I had planned of course but it did mean I knew how to be alert, aware and composed despite the carnage. Harrowing, dreadful and horrifying, but it was an experience. People can train, educate and theorise but it is experience that boosts the learning curve and forces you to think beyond what we are taught.

The turnaround

Three years from losing baby Edward, I fell pregnant again. It had been an agonising wait and not without panic. From all the physical trauma caused before, it was a concern as to whether a baby could 'stick' with all the scar tissue for a home. Of course every specialist flagged up my age. I was 44. That is senior in reproductive years but I was not going to let it get the better of me.

I was a ripe target for IVF and other 'assistance', and with every month of disappointment it could have been a temptation if there was more guarantee. But for my age group, hopes were low and the stakes were high. But tests showed that everything was healthy, balanced and working so I didn't want to risk chemical interference and blow my natural chances of conception. These tests even flattered me by resembling that of females 12 years my junior, a testament to mostly healthy living maybe?! But nonetheless, this pregnancy wasn't happening. My experience had taught me that a baby comes when it wants to, just as it leaves when it wants to, we're just their vehicle and maker … and this pregnancy was in no hurry.

The relief in a positive pregnancy test was huge but it was the start of a new worry. My son Oscar was six at the time and lectured me. He told me that I mustn't eat sugar and I must stop my dancing, 'especially those moves where you spin on your tummy, mummy'.

Although a healthy pregnancy, not a day passed without the fear of losing it. I wasn't being unduly negative, just mindful of and scarred by previous experiences. The elected C-section date came. I had exceptional surgeons, a private clinic and everything lined up for a positive outcome, yet the chilling fear of disaster pounced on me as I went to surgery. I caught the whole incision and process in the reflection of the aluminium lighting shades. The metal utensils being placed in tin trays was deafening and the smell of sterility all too reminiscent of death. But after rocking and pummeling, new life was held before my eyes. My girl stared me down with her icy blue eyes, it was a one-off look of pure intention, of soul-to-soul connection. She was here to stay.

Exercising

Because of my work, I had to remain active throughout my pregnancies, whether I felt like it or not. There were certainly times when I thought I'd faint from minimal exertion. I remember pacing through the woods, running with people while I was 5 months pregnant. We'd be plodding up a hill and panic set in as I couldn't draw the next breath and even when I did, it didn't satisfy recovery. I'd imposed pressure on myself that I mustn't let anyone down. Since I was the trainer, I couldn't be huffing and puffing flopped over a tree trunk! Instead, I would take off my rucksack, talk myself out of the panic and try to be as discreet as possible about my 'little turn'!

Although I am an advocate of exercising on an empty stomach (if only at easy to moderate intensity), things are very different while pregnant, and eating within a good time of rising will help avoid morning queasiness or even sickness.

So as a 'professional' I wouldn't encourage charging about at speed while pregnant! Not only for giddy reasons but for the extra weight and pressure put on the pelvis and its contents. We may well get away with it while pregnant and even during recovery after pregnancy, but think ahead a couple of decades or more and consider what condition you'd like to be in. Ration the impact now where possible.

Having had three Caesareans (two of which were emergency), plus the ruptured womb from one birth, long, high impact runs or similar are pretty much crossed off my repertoire of exercise. No matter the perfect surgery or attention to pelvic floor rehabilitation, I can see no reason to provoke further weakness to the pelvic region. There are plenty of women who have 'routine' procedures in fixing pelvic floor issues later in life, having had straightforward births, so it is a reminder that incontinence and other deterioration comes over time. Do what you can now to prevent such inconveniences in the future.

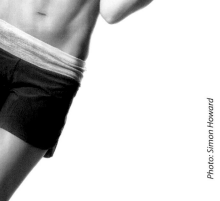

It is the nature of the constant pounding of running over a length of time that is of concern. Short sprints, hill climbs with walking in between will bring more benefits to heart, lungs and limbs anyway, so leave the long runs for just now and again.

As for postnatal exercises, there are a few types of classes and methods that cater for post birth recovery. Or so it seems. In the fitness industry it is easy to fall for the latest research and claims, but we have to remain discerning.

Photo: Simon Howard

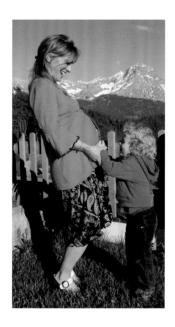

Research isn't always conducted as honestly as we trust and there are often oversights that are revealed later.

The important thing is that you are moving, encouraging circulation and releasing endorphins. Any resulting imbalances from the pregnancy and early months from carrying and feeding the newborn in awkward positions, can be helped with good osteopathic treatment. Once the alignment and structure is improved, look to gently build back strength with exercise, paying particular attention to the midsection area; the pelvic floor and lower back.

Post Caesarean and exercise

Anyone who has had a Caesarean will appreciate that just rolling over in bed and getting to the lavatory after surgery is an epic ordeal, so when it comes to gentle rehab exercises six weeks later, they just don't compare to the difficulty of trying to get out of bed! That doesn't mean to say you don't need them. Much of rehabilitating this corset of cut muscles is to start their education again, so as to avoid back pain later on.

And they cut deeply, through your abdominals, the transverses muscles and beyond. They also stretch, heave and rummage around. Just because it is a common procedure, does not mean it isn't a big operation. Ladies who have hysterectomies with the same method, need a good few weeks of recovery time. But a mum needs to be moving and nursing a baby within hours! So too much too soon can make for a set back later on.

Hurrying C-section recovery is futile. Walk, care for baby, care for the other children but don't push shopping trolleys or heave laundry baskets and vacuum cleaners around, that is where you need help. Getting back to exercise too soon will serve nothing. The progress in strengthening, fixing and shaping up is far more complete and faster if you leave those first 6 weeks to natural repair before starting an exercise programme. Resist any urge to perform most exercises other than walking.

The Caesarean scar itself can look rather messy to start with and it is hard to trust that within months, the red angry cut will be a neat white scar. Most likely there will be extra bump running above the cut, as if like a long thin sausage of flesh. Tight underwear that presses into the lower belly will temporarily encourage this sausage shape. With some surgical procedures in Asia and South America, they believe in compressing the area with tight bandage or bodice control style dressing. In Europe they hand out baggy surgical pants and leave it to you.

Over the first few months, this bulge does reduce though if fat weight is gained, it does return, looking more exaggerated. There is a fair amount of scar tissue and if C-sections are repeated, the bulky scar tissue may get chopped out for being obstructive while the surgeons are trying to access the baby. Still, all of this is nothing in the scheme of producing a baby safely.

Something that isn't really covered after surgery to this area is how you can feel a few months down the line. You are given rough guidelines about exercise and intercourse but the rest is up to you to find out. An aching back maybe one of the symptoms and it wouldn't be wrong to assume that this has something to do with reduced stomach muscle strength. The epidural's penetration into the spinal area is thought to leave niggling discomfort for quite a while. This becomes clear when following a good programme for not just strengthening the midsection (the lower back included), but mobilising it too, yet there is still backache.

Disconnected

Taking it a step further you may feel *disconnected* to your lower body, especially the pelvic region and its contents. It may sound far-fetched for the non-believer but the chi, energy, meridians, call it what you will, is really disrupted in this surgical procedure. We are normally caught up in our family role with the newborn to give it much thought, but for those practitoners who have equipment or skills in measuring this kind of energy, the evidence is unarguable. You only need to be reminded of peoples' accounts of losing a limb and the aches that remain in the void where the limb was, to appreciate the body has invisible energetic presence. Osteopathy can help, as can acupressure, acupuncture or un-invasive healing methods that you may feel inclined to try.

The first few weeks after baby arrives

This is the time when the vertical separation from chest to belly button, between the abdominals, can knit back together. This happens best alone, without any abdominal or core exercises in these initial weeks. It is very common to see the exercise obsessed types with a gap big enough to fit two fingers in, for years after baby. Some just never sealed up again due to overriding the natural pace of the body with an unsuitable or premature exercise plan. Wanting to shape up quickly can only worsen things. With every sit up or physical jerk, a bit of unprotected tummy squidges through the centre of the rib cage.

Exercises need to be executed slowly and accurately to start with. You have to get muscles and brain to 'reconnect' and this happens best with very primary exercises and breathing. Coughing and sneezing will give you a clear picture of where you

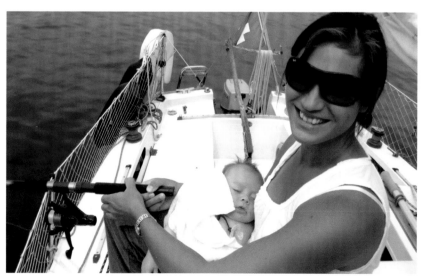

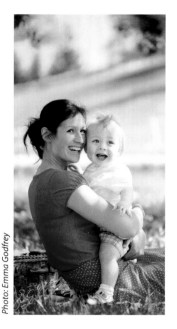

Photo: Emma Godfrey

are as far as a strong 'girdle' or core for a tummy. If it all blows up and trembles under the pressure of the cough or sneeze, there is basic work to be done to stabilise the area. Ideally, and it won't be straightaway, the tummy shouldn't need to move at all when we cough or sneeze.

Breastfeeding

Aside from the well-known benefits of breast feeding, while feeding from mum, the baby releases endorphins and becomes relaxed and comforted. There is no other consolation like mum's breast on a bad day. If feeding naturally becomes problematic then obviously the search for an appropriate alternative formula begins. It is likely that through the energy demanding process of making milk for the baby, that the metabolism is under higher demand and so using up maternal fat stores. Eating regularly and well (snacks included) ensure that you can get enough nutrients for both baby and you and also keeps the metabolism working well.

Keeping plates spinning!

I can't deny that I would rather work less and have more time to roll around on the floor playing with my children. But instead, like many of us, time is divided up by working, taking care of the family and the home. That is, without mentioning the dogs, bunny, garden and a husband who is frequently away.

Everyday has to be run to a tight timetable and seemingly concentrates on getting the basics done rather than reaching for the stars with adventures and high achievements. But it is the same for so many of us and we have to keep as many plates spinning simultaneously as possible.

Practical steps

Routine makes sure that the most important things happen: eating, son to school and dogs exercised. Lists take care of the rest, even if they do overflow and extend into the following day. But being able to handle the load efficiently without feeling overwhelmed, tired or fractious can be credited to good eating and self-care.

Even with a huge sleep debt, moods and energy are easily managed if the diet is right. Once you start feeding tiredness with pick-me-ups from starch and sugar, the battle begins and depletion slowly gets a hold.

No matter what, you must get a good balance of nutrients from your diet. Avocado, beansprouts, hemp seeds, fresh fruit, limes, kale and spinach are just a few of the 'must-have' foods throughout the week. A lacking diet leaves not just a de-mineralised and de-vitalised system, but one that is running ineffectively. This becomes all the more evident if you are breast feeding, so look out for yourself so that you can look out for your baby.

If you are on top of the eating side of things, getting on top of jobs will feel easier to work on. Something that really helps is blocking out and writing down times during the week where you can just focus and knuckle down with the 'must-dos'. It may only be 30 minutes here and there but it is a sure way to help you progress with a project, even if it is at reduced pace.

Splitting the time that you can find into *'Catching up'* days and *'key to success'* days helps separate the quagmire of tasks that need to be covered. Whole work days are ambitious and unlikely of course, but 30 minutes or maybe even an hour or two of uninterrupted, no distractions focus time, at least means that slowly but surely, things are achieved and projects can be realised. *'Catching up'* for me are things such as work correspondence, articles and sorting admin. They are not for desk clearing, getting caught up in social media, searching for cheap flights to Tahiti or wandering downstairs for another snack. *'Key to success'* slots are the things that really forge a plan on, in my case, filming mini workouts, setting up a fitness course ... *creating, making* and *marketing* moments.

So start by breaking down your jobs and goals. Then work out the steps to take to make them happen. Scribble them boldly into the diary into your **catching up** or **key to success** designated slots. That gives them importance and the reserved time they need for you to feel and know that you are moving ahead steadily.

The same goes for exercise. If it is written in the diary, it has much more chance of happening; otherwise it gets pushed to the end of the day and then ditched altogether. In summer, with the light mornings, getting up those few minutes earlier than the rest of the family feels easier and means that you can do a mini workout in just 10 minutes. The job, of course, is not to get distracted and start sifting through laundry or emptying the dishwasher. Admittedly dark mornings, after a bad night with crying infant, is tougher! Where we live, that early morning slot is taken up clearing snow off the steps, all 32 of them!

When my exercise routine has truly slipped, I go for a simple solution: one muscle group per day. There are two sets of weights on the landing, light and heavy. If between errands, nappy changing and anything else that crops up, I can pick up my weight and pull, press or squat for 30 seconds, I've got things rolling and muscle fibres working. A few mini gaps like that and a whole body part is worked out! It sounds sloppy and like it wouldn't be effective, but actually, so long as you fatigue that muscle, it will respond, whether it is in a snazzy spa gym or from flexing on the landing.

Waiting for a better opportunity is the first step to not getting started. So seize the moments where you can and there's no need for your pre-pregnancy body to be just a memory!

Tidy the Temple recipes

Emiko is one of the primary reasons this book exists. She came round one day and said what others had thought: this was an effective straightforward plan that had turned around many people's health and fitness and that I must share in book form with others.

It was just weeks after my baby, Edward, had died. I still don't know how I found the wherewithal or energy to write down all that I know with such enthusiasm and wholeheartedness so soon after such loss. But Emiko was instrumental in every part and laid out plans and deadlines while kindly encouraging me with her faith in my work and its results.

For both of us, the most important aspect was that you, the reader, gets honest and down-to-earth information, making this plan as achievable as possible and easy to commit to. The recipes are essential and the lists of food for the plan have had tremendous life put into them thanks to Emiko's inventions and modifications.

She knuckled down, creating and producing, and her diligence and attention inspired me. She produced dish after dish full of variety, tastes and textures that satisfy palate, tummy and, crucially, are easy to make. For months I had the pleasure of being the official tester and taster – dishes, drinks, samples and loaves all came my way. And I can promise you these recipes will not disappoint!

Eating is something of a hobby that Emiko and I share and, without hesitation, we agreed that puddings had to feature! Our 'Moving Forward' section provides a selection of nourishing breads, desserts and cakes that colour in 'healthy alternatives' in a way I've not encountered before.

I write without reservation that without Emiko's support and enthusiasm, I'd still be eating salmon and broccoli without a single chapter of this book completed.

Tidy the Temple is for you, me and anyone else who cares to make big, lasting changes without big effort.

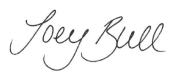

Tidy the Temple
RECIPES

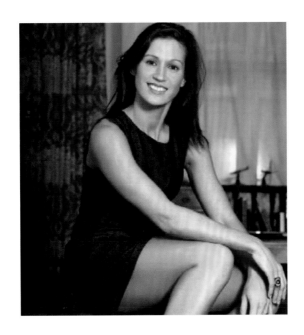

by Emiko Ray

J&E

www.tidythetemple.com

Thank yous

Thank you to:

my wonderful husband who always supports and believes in me and our fantastic boys Samson and Arthur who light up my life;

my other, fantastic 'A L P I N A' boys!

my fabulous mum and mother-in-law, who have educated me in the ways of Japanese and Vegetarian cuisine respectively;

Dad who always creates an air of excitement, expectation and delight around food;

Chieko for being such a STAR – you're amazing!

Andy for 'burning the candle at both ends' and for playing a big part in this project;

Amanda for being fab, fab, fab!

Sarah for your infinite nutritional wisdom and for EVERYTHING ELSE!

Dave, we cannot thank you enough for all you have done for us. You are such a good bloke;

Natalie and Anna for the way you have inspired me with your creative cooking;

Zany, Helen and Emma for your help. Zany-you are such a good sport!

Guy who has worked so hard for our cause;

Simon for being a talented and kind photographer!

Peter for your enthusiasm and hard work;

Julian, Daren and Andy at Tanner. What lovely people to work with;

A special thank you to my fun, generous, humble, and beautiful friend Joey, for making this all possible. *Tidy the Temple* is a fantastic course and something I am so proud to be a part of. Joey's commitment and passion for happy, healthy living is an example to us all.

Text copyright © 2013 Emiko Ray

Emiko Ray is hereby identified as the author of this work in accordance with the Copyright, Designs and Patents Act 1988.

All rights reserved. No part of this publication may be reproduced, stored in a retrieval system, or transmitted in any form or by any means, electronic, mechanical, photocopying, recording or otherwise without the prior permission of the copyright owner.

Photos of Emiko: Simon Howard. **Recipe photos:** Emiko Ray and Sarah Leo

ISBN: 9782839907149. Printed and bound in the UK by Butler Tanner & Dennis Ltd, Frome, Somerset.

First Published (2013) by J&E. www.tidythetemple.com

Part 2 *Tidy the Temple Recipes*

Contents

INTRODUCTION

The *Tidy the Temple* recipes are designed to make your 28 days and beyond as enjoyable and as stress-free as possible. However, even if you are not following the course, these recipes are a good foundation for healthy eating.

Tips for use

- **Some of the recipes are designed for later on in the plan,** so watch out for the added ingredients and pay attention to the food lists that follow.

- **The choice of foods is designed to reduce cravings, mobilise fat, clear out toxicity and to rev up the metabolism.** You may wonder why there are no grains, oats, brown rice or quinoa in the early stages. These are great foods but the first 28 days are about mobilising fat and fuelling our muscles. If losing fat is your goal then it won't matter that you may be eating more than before. The foods used in these recipes will assimilate well with your body and that is what matters. Try not to overcook food, especially vegetables; steaming is better.

- Chew your food thoroughly and do not eat in a hurry as this hinders digestion. If you were to eat fruit salad after a meat dish or most other food choices, you might feel bloated. For comfort, and to relieve the digestion, aim to eat in this order: fruit, carbohydrate, proteins.

- Do not re-freeze a dish that you have frozen previously.

- When making bread, try to buy slow-acting yeast.

- **Opt for good quality meats and pay attention to varying your protein choices.** Go for live organic yoghurt. Non-organic dairy cows can be supplemented with hormones, antibiotics and more. Goat and sheep yoghurt and cheese is also suggested.

- **Processed foods and anything with E numbers must GO!** If you don't understand the ingredients, don't buy it.

- **If you would like to make gluten and wheat free breads and desserts,** gluten and wheat free flour could be used in place of the flour suggested in the recipes and is easily accessible in shops and supermarkets. For the dessert section make sure the flour you use is ideal for either bread or cake-making. It should say on the packet.

- **Whilst cooking, feel free to experiment** with the range of oils mentioned in the list with the exception of flax oil. Use it as a dressing on salads or on food after cooking.

- **Where mirin is called for,** ensure you use good quality mirin with no added sugar or enzymes.

- **When using tempeh,** steam or grill it for 20 minutes. You can sprinkle over a little salt and fry it. Tempeh freezes well and keeps for approximately a week in the fridge in a zip-lock food bag. When it comes to thawing tempeh, steaming is good as well as thawing overnight in the fridge.

- **If you are trying to reduce your sugar intake** but still enjoy sweet treats then try some of the recipes by ensuring you use organic, pure cane sugar and simply reduce the amount of sugar suggested. As an alternative, use organic, unprocessed honey or organic pureed fruit.

- **Please photocopy or cut out the shopping list** at the back of the book to use when food shopping. You will also find the 'Helpful Tidy the Temple Recipe List' (p10) and 'Meal Planner' (p13) to aid you in food preparation.

- Standard level spoon measurements are used in all recipes. Measuring spoons (½ tsp, 1 tsp, 1 tbsp) will come in handy.

- **You will find a 'Notes' section with each recipe.** If you are anything like me, you will find this a helpful reminder of what you prepared as an accompaniment. Or, you may like to note who you shared the meal with (useful if you have a lot of people over for meals!) and if you changed the quantities.

- **I have used a fan-assisted oven** to prepare these recipes so please bear that in mind when cooking and baking.

- **When baking cakes** in the Moving Forward section, expect them to be a little heavier in consistency than you are perhaps used to. This is due to the fact that white flour and butter are not used.

Ratios and portions

Your plate needs a good balance of fibre and protein. Ensure that at least two thirds of the plate is salad and/or vegetables or fruit. The other third is protein. Keep this ratio the same for snacks. If you are a vegetarian you may need a half and half mix of vegetable protein and fibre. The same ratio will be good for snacks.

Don't concern yourself with portions for the first few days, it is the quality of food that matters now. It is much more beneficial to eat a full plate of food than not enough.

Recipe sections

28 DAY PLAN 'TIDY THE TEMPLE'

The 28 day plan for losing fat, toning up and boosting energy.

MOVING FORWARD

The 'Moving Forward Plan'. A healthy selection of recipes which can be used after the 28 day eating plan.

Happy cooking and bon appétit!

Food lists

List 1 *Food from Day 1*

PROTEINS: One to be eaten every meal

■ *HEAVIER PROTEINS* ■ *VEGETARIAN OPTIONS*

Cod	Crab	Haddock	Lobster	Mackerel
Monkfish	Prawns	Salmon	Sardines	Sea Bass
Shellfish	Sole	Swordfish	Tuna	
Beef	Chicken	Duck	Kidney	Lamb
Parma ham (with no added preservatives)	Pork	Turkey	Veal	All nuts
Chickpeas (tinned if necessary)	Eggs	Hemp seed	Houmous	Lentils
Seeds	Soya in moderation	Tempeh (fermented soybeans)		

FRUIT

Apples	Grapefruit	Lemons	Limes	Melon
Olives	Oranges	Pears	Pomegranates	

SALADS AND VEGETABLES

All leafy greens	All types of squash	Artichoke	Asparagus	Avocado
Aubergine	Broccoli	Cabbage (green and red)	Carrots	Cauliflower
Celery	Courgette	Cucumber	Fennel	*Fresh herbs:* parsley, basil, mint, sage, thyme etc.
Garlic	Ginger	Green beans	Kale	Leek
Mushroom	Onion and spring onion	Parsnip	Peas	Raw mung bean sprouts, all germinating seeds
Red and yellow pepper	Rocket	Seaweed	Spinach	Tomatoes

■ **A tasty tip:** Chop up a clump of your chosen herb, mix with some oil and ground nuts, season with salt and pepper, then sprinkle over meat, fish or vegetables to add some great flavour.

■ For a basic chicken and vegetable stock recipe see p57 in Joey's section.

■ Seasoning (sea salt and pepper) can be used freely. **Note:** Sea salt and pepper are not stipulated in the ingredients or shopping lists but ensure you have supplies at the ready!

OILS

Almond oil	Coconut oil	Flax oil	Hemp oil	Olive oil
Peanut oil	Sesame oil	Walnut oil		

■ When oil is heated, the composition and molecules change for the worse. Coconut oil is an exception and can be heated up to 170 degrees without any detrimental changes. Try to avoid overheating oils.

DRINKS

Coconut water	Freshly squeezed juice, homemade juices and smoothies (p14)	Fruit tea	Green tea	Herbal tea
Water				

List 2 *Food to introduce on Day 4*

FRUIT

Blueberries	Peaches	Pineapple	Raspberries	Strawberries

OTHER

All legumes, white and red kidney Beans	All spices and dry herbs	All pulses	Balsamic and apple cider vinegar	Live organic cow, sheep or goat yoghurt

List 3 *Food to introduce on Day 11*

FRUIT

Apricots	Blackberries	Blackcurrants	Cherries	Cranberries
Grapes	Plums	Redcurrants		

SALAD AND VEGETABLES

Beetroot	Radishes

GRAINS

Barley	Buckwheat	Millet	Oats

OTHER

Crunchy flaked soya (in moderation)	Smoked fish (e.g. salmon, mackerel)	Soy sauce (all natural ingredients)	Rice, oat, spelt and almond milk in moderation

List 4 *Food to introduce on Day 21*

FRUIT

Fresh figs

OTHER

Coconut	Coconut milk (natural)	Stock: if you prefer to buy stock, use one with all natural ingredients

List 5 *Food to introduce on Day 26*

GRAINS

Brown rice	Quinoa	Rye	Spelt

FLOURS

Barley	Buckwheat	Chestnut	Corn
Millet	Oat	Rye	Spelt

OTHER

Peanut/nut butter (all natural without hydrogenated fat)	Pumpernickel bread	Rye bread	Slow-acting yeast

Some fruits have more fructose than others, some taste sweeter and some have a higher glycemic index. Depending on an eating plan's approach, these factors and fruit choices, will vary in favour and may be confusing to the health conscious individual. Overall, eating more fruit in its fresh and raw state is always going to be much more beneficial than cooked, processed, pre-packaged or very acidic food. Tidy the Temple's goal is to tame the taste buds and so the majority of sweeter and softer fruits are introduced over time.

In List 3, to be introduced on Day 11, there are the following grains that can be introduced: Barley, buckwheat, oat and millet. By Day 26 and List 5, grains and flours feature more. Use these sparingly to avoid ending up in a carbohydrate heavy and over acidic eating plan. Try rotating carbohydrates and omitting on alternate days as suggested in daily message 11 and on page 147.

HELPFUL 'TIDY THE TEMPLE' RECIPE LIST

Make food preparation easy during the course by using the following list:

From Day 1

Aubergine Rolls	23
Baked Fish Fillet (without paprika)	50
Burgers (without dried herbs)	40
Carrot and Cucumber sticks with a Guacamole Dip	61
Carrot Soup (using homemade stock)	19
Courgette and Almonds	39
Fish Cakes with Cucumber Salsa (without yoghurt)	53
Fried Breakfast	15
Fried Fish	51
Grapefruit	15
Guacamole (without tabasco)	101
Herbal Tea	15
Houmous	101
Juices: '1', '2', '3'	14
King Prawn Salad (if fresh dill is used)	45
Lentil Salad	41
Lentil Soup (using homemade stock)	20
Lollies	54
Meat Balls (without dried herbs)	38
Melon	15
Melon with Parma Ham	24

Omelette (using fresh salmon)	15
Pea Soup (using homemade stock)	21
Ratatouille	44
Roast Chicken	33
Roasted Vegetables	52
Salmon with Cucumber and Pomegranate Salad (without paprika)	47
Sauce: Pesto	59
Scrambled Egg	15
Smoothies: 'Smooth', 'Refreshing', 'Filling', 'Creamy.'	14

Snacks — 61

- Dry seaweed shredded on top of a slice of tempeh
- Fruit and nuts
- Fruit with a slice of chicken
- Melon/Grapefruit sprinkled with hemp seed and almonds
- Stewed Orange (with a handful of prawns) — 54

From Day 4

From Day 11

From Day 21

From Day 26

'Tidy the Temple' Meal Planner

Photocopy this chart and plan your meals ahead

Monday	Tuesday	Wednesday	Thursday	Friday	Saturday	Sunday

BREAKFAST IDEAS
28 DAY PLAN

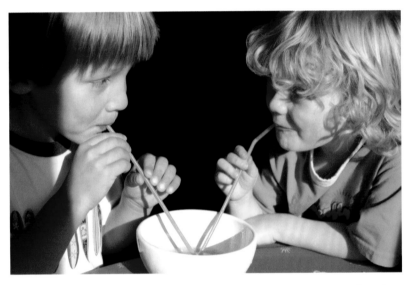

These recipes are generous in portions so you can share them with family and friends. Ensure you drink them just after preparing to benefit fully.

Smoothies and juices

Smoothies

Place the following ingredients in a blender or food processor:

Smooth	½ a grapefruit, 1 lime, 5 apples (or 120ml/4 fl oz organic apple juice)
Tangy	1 lemon, 1 lime, ½ small pineapple, 5 apples (or 120ml/4 fl oz organic apple juice)
Refreshing	1 apple, 2 oranges, 10 mint leaves
Filling	¼ of a cucumber, 10 mint leaves, 9 apples (or 220ml/7 fl oz organic apple juice to taste)
Sweet	½ a small pineapple, 1 lime, 5 apples (or 120ml/4 fl oz organic apple juice). Add ½ a grapefruit as a variation.
Creamy	½ a melon, 9 apples (or 220 ml/7 floz organic apple juice)

Juices

If you have a juice extractor, try the following juices:

'1' Juice	4 oranges, 1 apple and a large handful of lamb's lettuce
'2' Juice	3 apples, ½ a yellow pepper, 4 large lettuce leaves and a handful of mint
'3' Juice	4 oranges, 2 large carrots, 1 tsp of fresh ginger and a handful of mint

Smoothies and juices are a great way to start the day. They provide the body with nutrients and fast. Juices do not contain fibre and are, therefore, not as filling as smoothies which tend to use the whole fruit.

Some people prefer smoothies without the peel or pips but it really is personal preference.

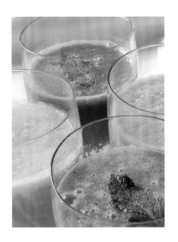

■ For more protein, try adding hemp or ground almonds to the smoothies and juices or choose something else from the protein list.

■ Experiment by adding a light sprinkling of mixed spice (e.g. nutmeg or cinnamon), or some herbal tea. Green tea which has been cooled in the fridge is a good choice.

Quick and tasty ideas

■ Drink some **herbal tea!** Green tea is great for giving you a boost first thing and it is full of antioxidants.

■ Cut a **grapefruit** in half and sprinkle ground almonds and hemp seed on top. Boil an egg too if you are hungry!

■ Eat half a **melon** with seeds and almonds.

■ **Fruit salad** including berries, with hemp (prepare a few portions in a pyrex dish with a lid and keep in the fridge).

■ Grill some **mackerel** and eat after some fruit.

■ **Scramble an egg** or two and eat with lightly heated cherry tomatoes.

■ **Fried breakfast** *Serves 1* Fry in a glug of olive oil 2 eggs, a handful of mushrooms and 4 cherry tomatoes.

■ **Fruit Parfait** *Serves 1* If you are using barley, first boil a handful in water for 40 minutes. In a dessert glass, chop a handful of fresh fruit and make layers of fruit and natural yoghurt. Sprinkle the top with either barley or oatflakes. Serve straight away.

■ **Omelette** *Serves 1* In a bowl, whisk an egg and add a small diced onion, a diced mushroom, some mint leaves, a few salmon streaks and some spinach leaves. Fry in a little olive oil for 3-5 minutes. (Use this for lunch/dinner as well. This is especially good for children – you can add goat's cheese to make it more interesting for them.)

REMEMBER

Just make sure you get protein and some vegetable and/or fruit.

If you are not an egg or nut eater, perhaps take fruit and slices of tempeh or one of the other proteins from the list.

You could even boil up lentils or chickpeas and be well prepared.

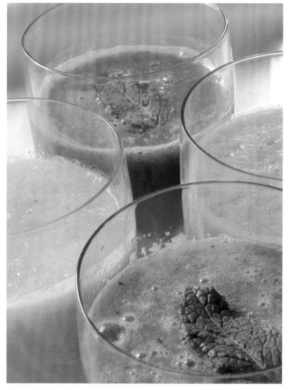

Smoothies

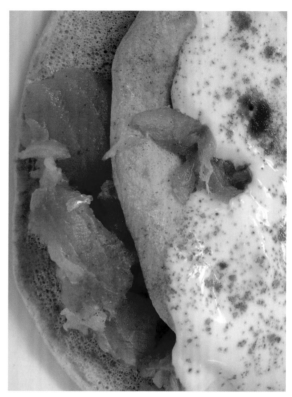

Buckwheat Pancakes

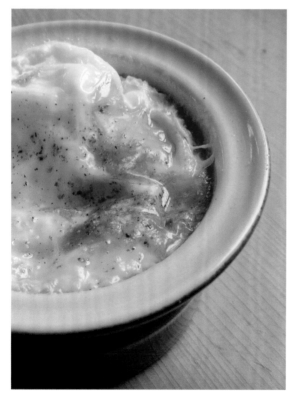

En Cocotte

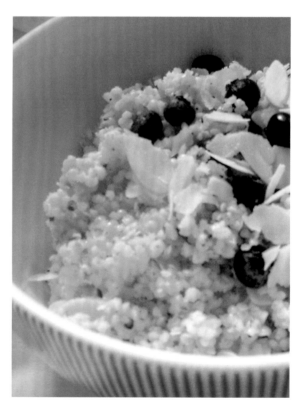

Millet Porridge

Buckwheat Pancakes

Makes 6. You can make these the night before.

1 Mix 100g/3 oz buckwheat flour, 1 egg, 300ml/11 fl oz cold water and ground pepper.

2 For each pancake, fry a ladleful of the mix in a little coconut oil.

3 Stack any left-overs in between cling film and freeze. You can fill them with: salmon and eggs; salmon, natural live yoghurt and a sprinkle of paprika; chicken and salad; watercress and avocado.

En Cocotte

Serves 1

1 Preheat the oven to 220°C/425°F/Gas Mark 7.

2 Rub the inside of a ramekin with olive oil and season with 1 tsp of freshly chopped thyme.

3 Add 2 tbsp of natural yoghurt.

4 Carefully break 2 eggs and place on top of the yoghurt.

5 Season with salt and pepper.

6 Put the ramekin into a small dish and pour water into the dish until it is half way up the sides of the ramekin.

7 Bake eggs until set and golden on top.

NOTES

Millet Porridge

Serves 2

1 Boil 300ml/11 fl oz water and add 75g/3 oz millet flakes (or buckwheat, barley or oat flakes).

2 Simmer for 5 minutes and serve with a mix of ground cinnamon, grated apple, hemp seed, berries, nuts or live yoghurt if you fancy.

3 Or add some rice, oat, spelt or almond milk instead of yoghurt, if desired.

LUNCH OR DINNER IDEAS 28 DAY PLAN

Butternut Squash Soup (V)

Ingredients *Serves 4*

1.5kg/3.3lbs butternut squash

2 tbsp olive oil

1 onion

2 garlic cloves

1 tsp nutmeg

¼ tsp curry powder

240ml/8 fl oz freshly squeezed apple juice (approx 2 large apples)

NOTES

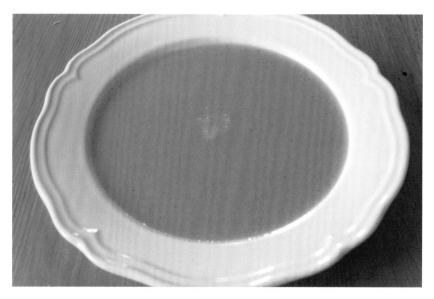

This soup is easy, tasty and filling.

1   Heat 2 tbsp of olive oil in a large saucepan over a medium heat.

2   Fry 1 chopped onion for about 2 minutes. Stir in 2 chopped garlic cloves, ¼ tsp of curry powder and 1 tsp of nutmeg.

3   Add 1.5kg/3.3lbs peeled and diced butternut squash. Cook for 6 to 8 minutes, stirring occasionally. Stir in 950ml/33 fl oz water. Bring to the boil and then reduce heat. Simmer for about 20 minutes until the squash is tender.

4   Remove from the heat and blend the contents of pan until smooth. Transfer back to the pan and add 1 tsp of salt and 240ml/8 fl oz freshly squeezed apple juice (approx. the juice of 2 large apples). Stir well before serving.

Tips: Add water to suit your preferred soup consistency.
Freeze any soup you do not use in separate freezer bags.

Carrot Soup (V)

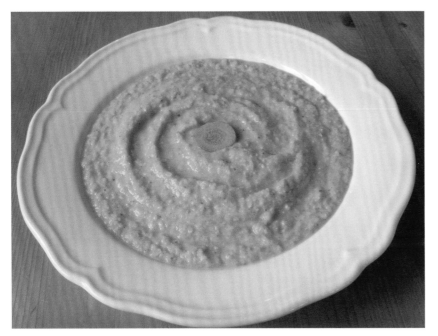

Ingredients *Serves 4*

2 onions

2 garlic cloves

6 carrots

2 celery stalks

1 tbsp natural veg stock powder

herbs of your choice

100g/4 oz ground almonds

The sweetness of the carrots make this soup utterly delicious!

1 Peel and chop 2 onions, 2 garlic cloves, 6 carrots and 2 celery stalks. Put into a saucepan with 900ml/32 fl oz hot vegetable stock (using 1 tbsp of natural vegetable stock powder).

2 Cover the pan and bring to the boil, adding some herbs of your choice.

3 Lower the heat and simmer until the vegetables are soft, then stir in 100g/4 oz ground almonds.

4 Blend the contents of pan until smooth.

Tips: *Add water to suit your preferred soup consistency.*
      Freeze any soup you do not use in separate freezer bags.

NOTES

Lentil Soup (V)

Ingredients *Serves 4*

200g/7 oz puy lentils

2 tbsp natural veg stock powder

1 onion

100g/4 oz spinach leaves

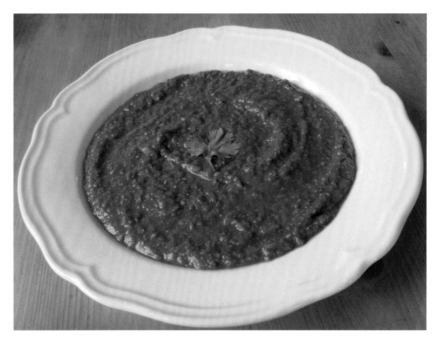

A hearty filling soup– a real winter warmer.

NOTES

1 Boil 200g/7 oz lentils for 30 minutes with 900ml/32 fl oz hot vegetable stock (using 2 tbsp of natural vegetable stock powder).

2 Place a diced onion and 100g/4 oz of spinach leaves into a steamer.

3 Place the steamer on top of the lentil pan and steam the vegetables until the lentils are ready.

4 Remove from the heat and blend the vegetables with the lentils and stock until smooth. After the 28 day plan, you can add marmite for extra flavour.

Tips: Add water to suit your preferred soup consistency.
Freeze any soup you do not use in separate freezer bags.

Pea Soup (V)

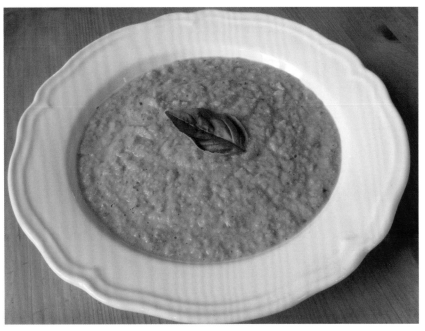

Ingredients *Serves 4*

5 tbsp olive oil

2 large onions

1 celery stick

1 carrot

1 garlic clove

400g/14 oz frozen peas

1 tbsp natural veg stock powder

25g/1 oz fresh basil leaves

The pea and basil really work well together to give this soup a sweet and fresh vibe!

1 Heat 5 tbsp of olive oil in a large saucepan.

2 Peel and chop 2 large onions, 1 celery stick, 1 carrot and 1 garlic clove and place into the saucepan.

3 Cover the pan and cook over a low heat until the vegetables are soft, stirring occasionally.

4 Add 400g/14 oz frozen peas and 900ml/32 fl oz hot vegetable stock (using 1 tbsp of natural vegetable stock powder).

5 Add 25g/1 oz fresh basil leaves if desired and simmer for 10 minutes.

6 Remove from the heat and blend until smooth.

Tips: Add water to suit your preferred soup consistency.
Freeze any soup you do not use in separate freezer bags.

NOTES

Mixed Vegetable & Coconut Milk Soup (V)

Ingredients *Serves 4*

1 clove garlic

1 onion

4 carrots

1 beetroot

glug of olive oil

240g/8 oz frozen peas

½ cauliflower

2 bay leaves

handful fresh coriander

1 tbsp natural veg stock powder

240ml/8 fl oz coconut milk

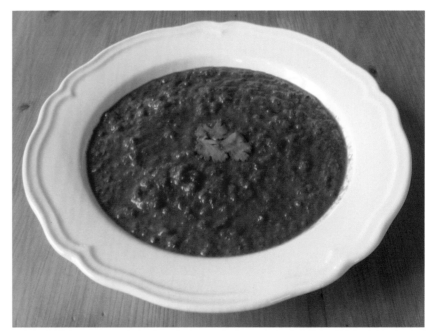

Don't let the colour put you off! This soup is a real winner.

NOTES

1 Peel and chop 1 clove garlic, 1 onion, 4 carrots, 1 beetroot (peeled and diced) and fry in a large saucepan with a glug of olive oil.

2 Add 240g/8 oz frozen peas, ½ a chopped cauliflower head, 2 bay leaves, 1 tsp of salt, a sprinkle of pepper and a handful of freshly chopped coriander.

3 Add 800ml/28 fl oz hot vegetable stock (using 1 tbsp of natural vegetable stock powder).

4 Cover the pan and bring to the boil. Lower the heat and simmer until the vegetables are soft.

5 Five minutes before removing the pan from the heat, add 120ml/4 fl oz of coconut milk. Remove the bay leaves and blend.

6 Add another 120ml/4 fl oz coconut milk after blending.

Tips: Add water to suit your preferred soup consistency.
Freeze any soup you do not use in separate freezer bags.

Aubergine Rolls (V)

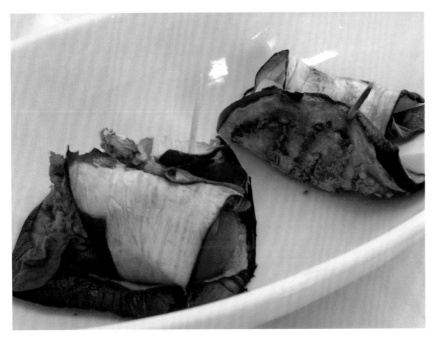

The tomato and basil duo are simply delicious.

Ingredients *Makes 10*

1 aubergine

glug of olive oil

10 basil leaves

100g/1.75 oz tempeh

10 cherry tomatoes

1 Slice thin strips off 1 whole aubergine, sprinkle salt over the slices and leave to sweat.

2 Turn and repeat.

3 Place the strips on foil, on a baking tray and brush with olive oil.

4 Grill until a little bronzed, then repeat on the other side.

5 Place a basil leaf, a small chunk of tempeh (fried in salt and olive oil beforehand) and a cherry tomato on to each aubergine strip and roll up, securing with a toothpick.

6 Grill for a further 5 minutes.

7 Season with salt and pepper before serving. Mince meat can also be used inside, instead of tempeh. Put any left-overs in the fridge and heat up the next day, for a snack.

NOTES

Melon with Parma Ham

Ingredients *Serves 4.*
A good starter.

8 slices parma ham

1 melon (galia, cantaloupe, watermelon or a selection of all three)

80g rocket

1 pomegranate

glug of olive oil

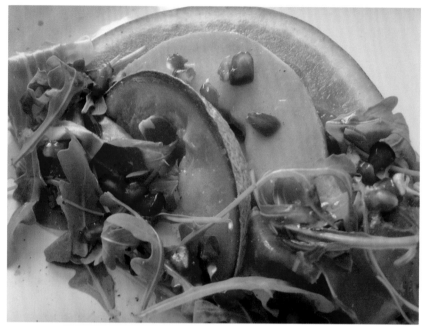

A selection of melon pieces coupled with a sprinkle of pomegranate seeds makes this stand out from your regular 'Melon with Parma Ham'.

NOTES

Repeat this for each plate:

1   Cut the melon into thin slices. Arrange on the plate.

2   Place 2 slices of parma ham over the melon slices.

3   Arrange a few rocket leaves over the melon and parma ham.

4   Scatter a few pomegranate seeds on top.

5   Finish with a glug of olive oil and a dash of freshly ground pepper.

Eggy Bread (V)

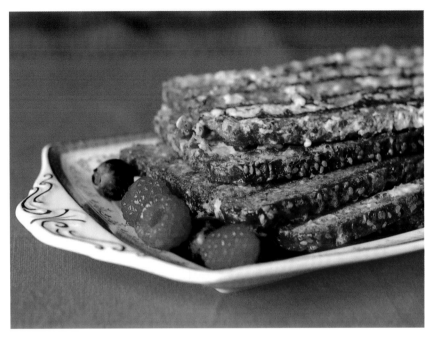

Ingredients *Serves 1*

glug of olive oil

1 egg

50ml/2 fl oz rice milk

1 or 2 slices rye or pumpernickel bread

Slices of fresh fruit of your choice

(honey)

Eggy bread used to feature alot growing up. Mum made the best Eggy Bread on a Saturday morning.

1 Brush a griddle pan with olive oil and heat.

2 Mix one egg and 50ml/2 fl oz rice milk in a wide bowl.

3 Place one or two slices of rye or pumpernickel bread and soak both sides. (See page 97 for a rye bread recipe).

4 Place the coated bread in the pan and fry until golden brown. Turn and fry the other side.

5 Serve with fruit and/or *honey (*honey after the 28 day plan).

Tip: *You want to fry this until you get a nice and soft inside with a slightly crunchy outside.*

NOTES

Grilled Tomatoes (V)

Ingredients *Serves 1*

glug of olive oil

1 large tomato

1 slice rye or pumpernickel bread

drizzle balsamic vinegar

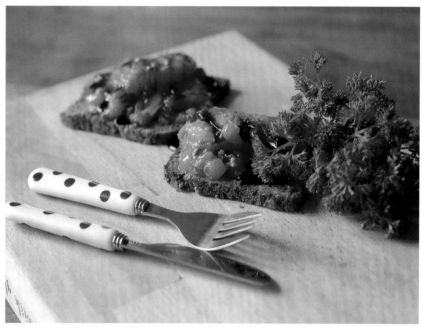

So quick and easy!

NOTES

1 Brush a griddle pan with olive oil.

2 Add thick slices of tomatoes and cook for 4 minutes.

3 Turn once until softened.

4 Arrange on a slice of rye or pumpernickel bread and drizzle with olive oil and balsamic vinegar. (See page 97 for a rye bread recipe).

Soy Mung Bean Sprouts (V)

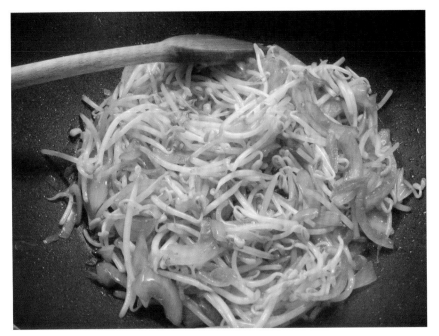

This is such a useful side dish to many meals.

Ingredients *Serves 2*

2 tbsp olive oil

1 tbsp soy sauce

200g/7 oz raw mung bean sprouts

1 tsp sesame oil

1 large onion

1 Slice one large onion thinly and fry in 2 tbsp of olive oil until soft.

2 Add 1 tbsp of soy sauce and 200g/7 oz mung bean sprouts and cook for a few minutes (not too long).

3 Add 1 tsp of sesame oil and serve immediately.

NOTES

Thai Curry with Tempeh and Vegetables (V)

Ingredients *Serves 1*

glug of olive oil

1 small onion

1 garlic clove

2 tsp curry powder

handful fresh basil

2 handfuls fresh coriander

415ml/15 fl oz coconut milk

½ broccoli head

½ red pepper

100g/3.5 oz tempeh

2 lime wedges

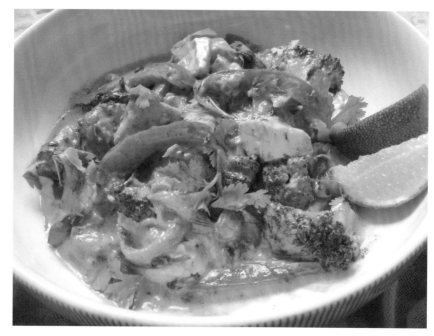

This healthy curry is super filling and tasty. Chicken can be used as an alternative to tempeh. Don't forget the lime wedges and coriander.

NOTES

1 Fry 1 small chopped onion (halved lengthwise and sliced crosswise) in a glug of olive oil for 3 minutes on a high heat. Stir occasionally.

2 Reduce to a moderate heat and add 1 crushed garlic clove, 2 tsp of curry powder and a handful each of freshly chopped basil and coriander. Cook for a further minute.

3 Stir in 415ml/15 fl oz coconut milk, 1 tsp of salt and 60ml/2 fl oz water and bring to the boil.

4 Stir in ½ chopped head of broccoli and ½ a sliced red pepper and bring to the boil.

5 Cover the pan and reduce the heat to a simmer, stirring occasionally for 2 minutes.

6 Gently stir in 100g/3.5 oz of tempeh (cut into ½ inch cubes) and cook for 20 minutes until the vegetables are tender, with the pan partially covered.

7 Serve with lime wedges and a handful of fresh coriander.

Nutty Mixed Salad (V)

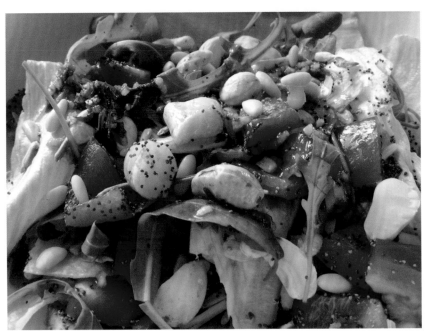

This is such a useful side dish to many meals … filling and tasty.

Ingredients *Serves 1*

2 large lettuce leaves

handful rocket

¼ pepper

1 radish

4 cherry tomatoes

½ thumb size spring onion

handful cashews, pine nuts, sunflower and poppy seeds

2 brazil nuts

Salad dressing Ingredients

1 tbsp soy sauce

1 small garlic clove

1 tbsp olive oil

sprinkle parsley

1 Throw together 2 large lettuce leaves, a handful of rocket, ¼ of a chopped pepper, 1 sliced radish, 4 halved baby tomatoes, half a thumb-size of spring onion, sliced, and 2 chopped brazil nuts.

2 Add a handful of cashew nuts and poppy seeds, and a sprinkle of sunflower seeds and pine nuts. Add …

3 *Salad Dressing (V):* 1 tbsp of soy sauce, 1 small garlic clove (crushed), 1 tbsp of olive oil and a sprinkle of chopped parsley. After the 28 day plan, you can add 1 tsp of mustard to the dressing.

NOTES

Millet Cauliflower (V)

Ingredients *Serves 2*

150g/5 oz millet

1 tbsp natural veg stock powder

1 small cauliflower head

2 garlic cloves

1 tsp each ground cumin, paprika and curry powder

handful fresh parsley

1 large red onion

60g/2 oz frozen peas

1 dollop natural yoghurt

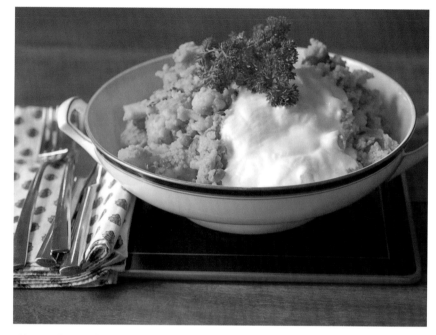

Gluten-free millet is high in fibre. If you are feeling a little stressed today, try this dish; the serotonin in millet is known to have a calming affect.

NOTES

1 Wash 150g/5 oz millet well in water and drain. Place in a large saucepan.

2 Add 500ml/18 fl oz hot vegetable stock (using 1 tbsp of natural vegetable stock powder).

3 Add 1 small chopped cauliflower, 2 crushed garlic cloves, 1 tsp of ground cumin, 1 tsp of paprika, 1 tsp of curry powder, ½ tsp of salt, 60g/2 oz frozen peas, a handful of freshly chopped parsley and 1 large chopped onion. Stir to mix.

4 Add 100ml/4 fl oz water. Bring to the boil and then turn down the heat.

5 Cover and simmer for about 25 minutes, stirring occasionally, until stock has reduced but is still a little stodgy in texture.

6 Serve with a large dollop of natural yoghurt and some fresh parsley. Finish with a sprinkle of paprika.

Stuffed Tomatoes

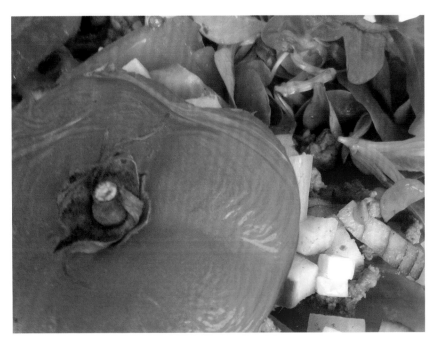

Ingredients *Serves 2*

2 large, relatively firm beef tomatoes

½ courgette

½ yellow pepper

½ onion

¼ cucumber

1 tbsp lemon juice

1 tbsp coriander

1 tbsp olive oil

1 tbsp curry powder

1 tbsp cumin seeds

250g/9 oz beef mince

1 tbsp natural beef stock powder

This dish needs slightly more prep than some of the other recipes but this looks really good when it is on the plate and tastes great too!

1 Preheat the oven to 200°C/400°F/Gas Mark 6. Cut off the tops of 2 relatively firm, large beef tomatoes and put to one side. Scoop out the tomato pulp, dice and place in a bowl.

2 Season the tomato shells with salt and pepper and turn them upside down on absorbent kitchen paper.

3 Dice ½ a courgette, ½ a yellow pepper, ½ an onion and add to the tomato pulp. Add 1 tbsp of lemon juice, 1 tbsp of freshly chopped coriander, 1 tbsp of olive oil, 1 tbsp of curry powder and 1 tbsp of cumin seeds. Stir well.

4 Cook 250g/9 oz minced beef with 100ml/4 fl oz beef stock (using 1 tbsp of natural beef stock powder). Add the beef to the pulp, stir well.

5 Place the mixture into the tomato skins. Add a dash of salt and pepper, place the tops on the tomatoes.

6 Put the tomatoes in an oiled roasting tin and heat for 20 minutes until cooked. Serve with a ¼ diced cucumber sprinkled over the stuffing. Drain excess juice and serve.

NOTES

Stuffed Squash

Ingredients *Serves 2.*
This is a variation of
Stuffed Tomatoes.

1 butternut squash or pumpkin

½ courgette

½ yellow pepper

½ onion

1 tbsp lemon juice

1 tbsp olive oil

1 tbsp curry powder

1 tbsp cumin seeds

250g/9 oz beef mince

1 large tomato

handful mint leaves

sprinkle flaked soya

NOTES

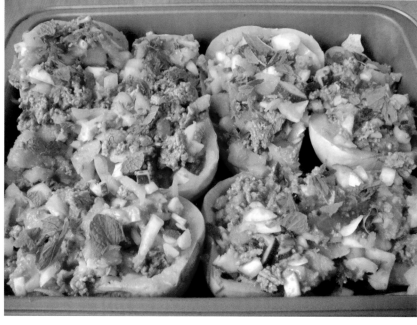

This dish is really filling and a firm favourite in our household!

1   Preheat the oven to 200°C/400°F/Gas Mark 6. Place one squash in an oiled roasting tin and put it in the oven for 30 minutes until softened.

2   When the squash is ready, cut it in half and discard the seeds (a grapefruit spoon is particularly effective). Take the pulp out of the skin and place into a big bowl, paying attention not to scoop too close to the edges otherwise the sides will collapse.

3   Dice ½ a courgette, ½ a yellow pepper, ½ an onion and add to the bowl. Add 1 tbsp of lemon juice, 1 tbsp of olive oil, 1 tbsp of curry powder and 1 tbsp of cumin seeds. Stir well.

4   Fry 250g/9 oz beef mince. When the beef is cooked, add 1 large diced tomato, stir and then turn off the heat.

5   Add the beef and tomato to the bowl and stir well. Place the mixture back into the squash skins. Add a sprinkle of salt and pepper. Cook in the oiled roasting tin for about 20 minutes and then add some freshly chopped mint leaves. If you have any left over pulp, sprinkle some flaked soya on top and place in an oven proof dish. Cook in the oven with the squash.

Roast Chicken

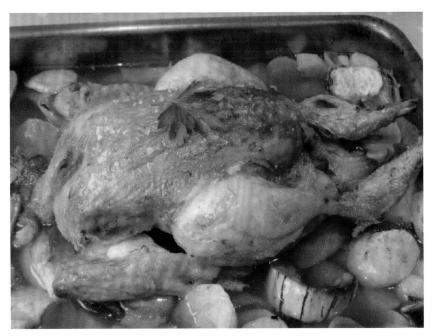

Ingredients *Serves 4*

1 large chicken

1 lemon

5 garlic cloves

glug of olive oil

a few parsnips, onions, carrots and leeks

I really haven't come across an easier way to cook a roast chicken … add any other root veg that takes your fancy and you won't be disappointed.

1 Preheat the oven to 180°C/350°F/Gas Mark 4.

2 Stuff a chicken with 1 lemon cut into quarters.

3 Add 2 garlic cloves, salt and pepper.

4 Drizzle a generous glug of olive oil over both sides of the chicken and season well with salt and pepper.

5 Rub one crushed clove of garlic into the olive oil on both sides of the chicken.

6 Chop parsnips, leeks, onions and carrots. Place under and around the chicken in a roasting tray.

7 Add 2 crushed garlic cloves, salt, pepper and a splash of olive oil. Pour some water over the vegetables until they are just covered.

8 Roast the chicken for 1 hour 20 minutes. After 50 minutes turn the chicken over in the tray and stir the vegetables.

9 To thicken the gravy, blend some of the vegetables and mix them back in with the juices. If you use a small chicken, cook for 1 hour only.

NOTES

Chicken Tikka

Ingredients *Serves 1.*
Prepare the chicken overnight.

1 chicken breast

300g/11 oz natural yoghurt

1 garlic clove

sprinkle tandoori, tikka or curry powder

For soy spinach

50g/2 oz pine nuts

1 garlic clove

olive oil

2 handfuls fresh spinach

1 tbsp soy sauce

NOTES

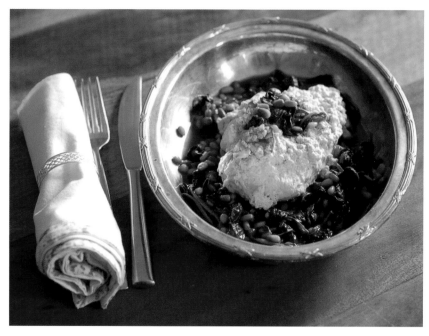

I really like the combination of the spinach and chicken in this.

1   Mix 300g/11 oz natural yoghurt with 1 crushed garlic clove, some ground pepper and either a sprinkle of tandoori, tikka or curry powder to marinate 1 chicken breast.

2   Leave in the fridge overnight or if you are in a hurry, a couple of hours will do, and cook in a dish, in the oven, for 12 minutes (using all the marinade) at 240°C/464°F/Gas Mark 9. Serve with **soy spinach.**

3   *To make the soy spinach (V).* Fill ⅔ of the bottom of a pan with pine nuts and fry with 1 crushed garlic clove and a glug of olive oil. When the pine nuts are brown, throw in two handfuls of fresh spinach, add 1 tbsp of soy sauce and cook until the spinach has reduced in size slightly.

Green Indian Chicken Curry

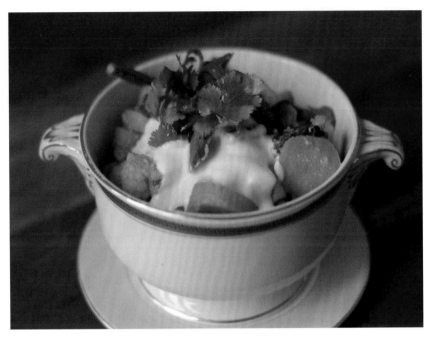

A great evening meal. The yoghurt, coriander and toasted almonds finish this dish off so well.

Ingredients *Serves 1*

1 chicken breast (or beef/lamb as an alternative)

1 small onion

1 garlic clove

1 tsp each ground turmeric, ground coriander, ground paprika and ground cumin

¼ cauliflower head

small handful green beans

2 carrots

2 tbsp ground almonds

small handful fresh spinach

fresh coriander

dollop natural yoghurt

handful flaked almonds

glug of olive oil

1 Fry 1 small diced onion and 1 chopped garlic clove in a generous glug of olive oil.

2 When the onions have softened, add 1 tsp each of ground turmeric, ground coriander, ground paprika, ground cumin and cook, stirring frequently for a minute or two.

3 Add 1 chicken breast cut into chunks and coat in the spice mix. Brown the chicken.

4 Add ¼ of a cauliflower head cut into small florets, a small handful of green beans and 2 carrots (peeled and coarsely chopped). When these are coated in the mixture, add 225ml/8 fl oz boiling water. Stir well.

5 Add 2 tbsp of ground almonds and a small handful of spinach and simmer for about 20 minutes until the carrots are cooked through and the chicken is tender. Add more water to the sauce if needed.

6 Sprinkle some fresh coriander over the curry and serve with a dollop of natural yoghurt and a scattering of toasted almonds. Use beef or lamb as an alternative.

NOTES

Soy Steak

Ingredients *Serves 1*

1 sirloin steak

glug of olive oil

2 garlic cloves

3 tbsp soy sauce

4 mushrooms

1 onion

serve with broccoli or Nutty Mixed Salad (p29)

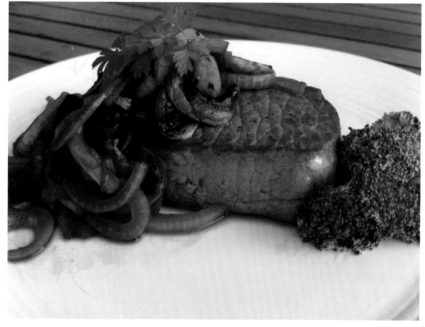

I LOVE this. Quick, easy and very tasty.

NOTES

1 Marinate 1 sirloin steak in olive oil and 2 crushed garlic cloves for 15 minutes.

2 Place the steak into a large pan on high heat. Add the remaining marinade and 3 tbsp of soy sauce. Cook the steak until the juice starts coming out. Be careful not too overcook this delicious meat.

3 Dice 4 mushrooms and 1 onion and add to the juice.

4 Serve topped with the mushroom and onion mix on top.

5 If the meat is ready before the vegetables, set the meat aside in a heat-proof dish while the vegetables cook. Serve immediately with steamed broccoli or *Nutty Mixed Salad (V) (page 29)*.

Moroccan Beef Stew with Pumpkin

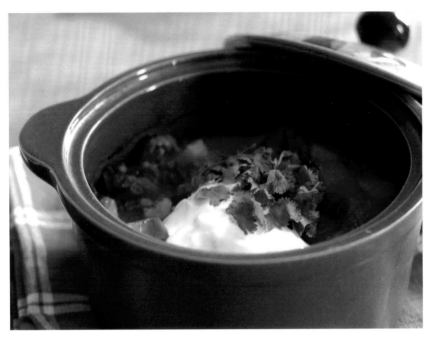

The pumpkin and plums make this dish.

Ingredients *Serves 2*

glug of olive oil

1 large onion

1 garlic clove

2 tsp ground cumin

250g/9 oz stewing beef

2 ripe tomatoes

200g/7 oz pumpkin (or butternut squash)

1 tbsp natural beef stock

1 bay leaf

3 large roughly chopped plums

2 tbsp ground almonds

fresh coriander

dollop of natural yoghurt

1 Preheat the oven to 170°C/325°F/Gas Mark 3.

2 On the hob, heat a good glug of olive oil in a large non-stick pan.

3 Gently fry 1 large chopped onion and 1 finely chopped garlic clove.

4 Add 2 tsp of ground cumin and fry for a minute or two.

5 Add 250g/9 oz (stewing) beef and coat the beef in the mixture turning regularly until just browned.

6 Add 2 ripe chopped tomatoes and bring to the simmer.

7 Add 200g/7 oz pumpkin, or butternut squash (skinned, seeded and cut into chunks), 250ml/8 fl oz hot beef stock (using 1 tbsp of natural beef stock powder), 1 bay leaf and a sprinkle of salt and pepper.

8 Simmer, then add 3 large roughly chopped plums and 2 tbsp of ground almonds.

9 Transfer to a casserole dish, cook for an hour or until the beef is tender.

10 When ready to serve, sprinkle with a generous amount of chopped coriander and a dollop of natural yoghurt.

NOTES

Meat Balls

Ingredients *Makes 6 balls.*

250g/9 oz beef mince

1 red onion

3 garlic cloves

2 tsp dried mixed herbs

3 good sized tomatoes

pinch paprika

12 basil leaves

serve with steamed vegetables or Courgette and Almonds (p39)

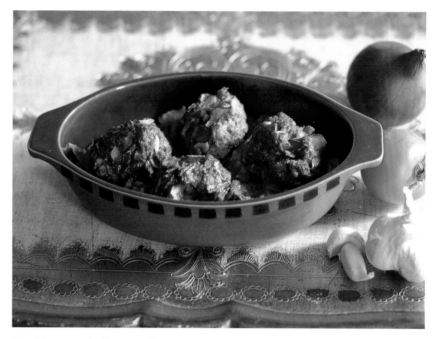

Healthy meatballs served in a tomato sauce. I have a thing for basil but this meal really benefits from those basil leaves.

NOTES

1   Preheat the oven to 180°C/350°F/Gas Mark 4.

2   Blend 250g/9 oz of beef mince, ½ of the chopped red onion, 6 chopped basil leaves, 2 crushed garlic cloves, 1 tsp of dried mixed herbs and a dash of salt and ground pepper, until smooth.

3   Shape the mixture into balls and chill in the fridge for 30 minutes.

4   In a saucepan, lightly fry the rest of the chopped red onion, 1 crushed garlic clove, 3 good-sized chopped tomatoes, a pinch of paprika, 1 tsp of dried mixed herbs and 6 chopped basil leaves. Add a little water in the pan to thicken the tomato sauce (if needed) and simmer for 15 minutes.

5   Transfer the sauce to an ovenproof dish and arrange the meatballs on top. Cook in the oven on the middle shelf for 30 minutes and serve with steamed vegetables or **Courgette and Almonds (V)** (page 39).

Courgette and Almonds (V)

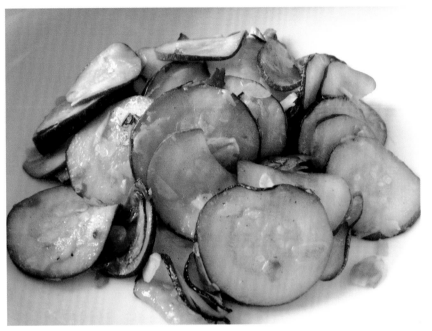

Ingredients *Serves 2*

2 handfuls flaked almonds

glug of olive oil

1 courgette

1 or 2 garlic cloves

(1 onion)

This reminds me of holidays in France. Mother of six, Zilla, never ceases to amaze me with her 'calm', her cooking and this most wonderful side dish.

1   Toast 2 handfuls of flaked almonds in a hot pan with a glug of olive oil and a sprinkle of salt, stirring until slightly browned.

2   Add 1 finely sliced courgette with 1 or 2 crushed garlic cloves, according to taste and cook until soft and slightly browned.

3   Chop and fry 1 onion with the courgette if you want to bulk out the dish.

Tip: *Be patient when cooking those courgettes. They will turn brown eventually but don't let them burn to a crisp! This is a fab side dish.*

NOTES

Burgers

Ingredients

Makes 4 burgers.

250g/9 oz beef mince

1 onion

glug of olive oil

sprinkle of dried Italian herbs

fresh coriander

1 egg

serve with Lentil Salad (p41) or Ginger Garlic Green Beans (p42)

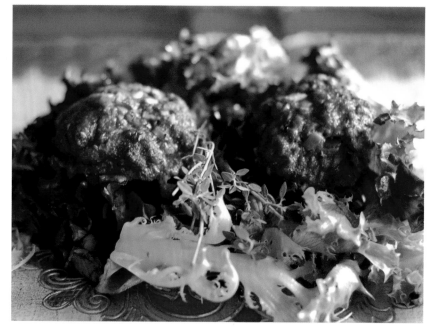

Simple burgers. Don't buy them pre-packed as they are really easy to make.

NOTES

1 Preheat the oven to 180°C/350°F/Gas Mark 4.

2 Place 250g/9 oz of minced beef in a bowl.

3 Fry 1 finely chopped onion gently in a glug of olive oil.

4 Add ground pepper, a sprinkle of dried Italian herbs, freshly chopped coriander, and the fried onion into the bowl. (You can add 1 tbsp of tomato purée after the 28 day plan).

5 Mix altogether with 1 raw whisked egg and shape into burgers.

6 Place in fridge for 30 minutes then cook for 30 minutes on the middle shelf, on a greased baking tray.

7 Serve with *Lentil Salad (V) (page 41)* or *Ginger Garlic Green Beans (page 42).*

   Tip: *Once made, like the meat balls, these will need to chill for 30 minutes in the fridge.*

Lentil Salad (V)

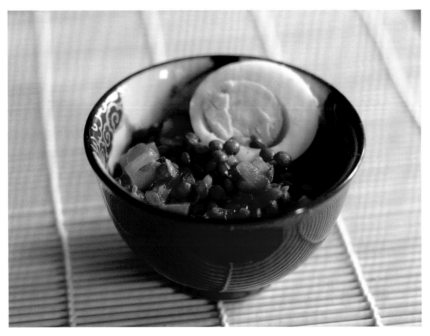

Ingredients *Serves 1*

50g/2 oz puy lentils

½ red onion

1 tbsp olive oil

1 large tomato

1 lime

4 or 5 basil leaves

1 egg

I love the lime in this Lentil Salad. This is one of Joey's favourites she cooks up for me. Great to dress up any meal or just to eat all on its own.

1   Boil 50g/2 oz of Puy lentils in 500ml/18 fl oz water for 30 minutes.

2   In a pan, fry ½ a finely chopped red onion in 1 tbsp of olive oil until soft and then take off the heat.

3   Add 1 chopped tomato to the pan and grate the skin of 1 lime over the onions.

4   Add the juice of ½ the lime to the pan and 4 or 5 freshly chopped basil leaves.

5   Add the drained lentils to the pan and simmer for a further 2 minutes.

6   Add a couple of slices of boiled egg just before serving. You can also use chickpeas as an alternative to lentils.

NOTES

Ginger Garlic Green Beans

Ingredients *Serves 4*

500g/18 oz green beans

2 tbsp olive oil

1 tsp sesame oil

2 garlic cloves

2.5cm/1 inch fresh ginger

1 tbsp natural chicken stock powder

2 tbsp soy sauce

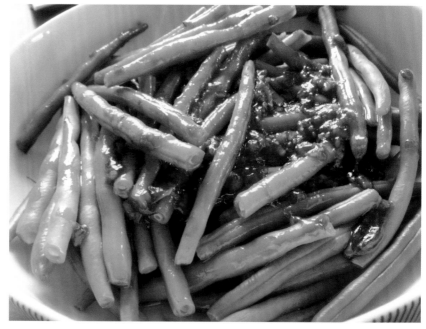

This is a great sauce for the green beans. Just make sure you keep stirring stirring stirring …

NOTES

1 Chop the ends off 500g/18 oz of green beans and steam over a saucepan of boiling water for about 5 minutes, until tender.

2 Heat 2 tbsp of olive oil, 1 tsp of sesame oil and 2 crushed cloves of garlic for 2 minutes.

3 Stir in 2.5cm/1 inch fresh ginger (peeled and thinly sliced), 1 tbsp of natural chicken stock powder and 2 tbsp of soy sauce, stirring constantly for 2 minutes.

4 Pour the mixture over the beans and serve immediately.

Red Bean Burger (V)

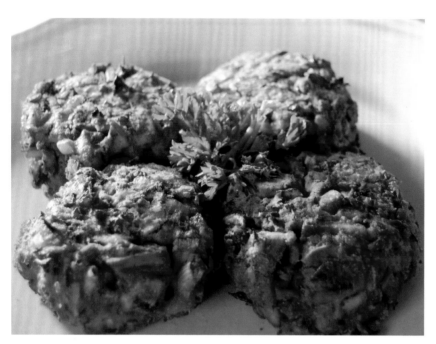

Ingredients
Makes 4 burgers.

1 tbsp olive oil

1 small onion

1 garlic clove

1 tsp each of ground cumin, ground coriander and ground turmeric

115g/4 oz mushrooms

400g/14 oz kidney beans (or a can)

serve with salad or Ratatouille (p44)

My friend Anna made this at one of her BBQs and and it was a great hit with the non-vegetarians and vegetarians alike.

1 Preheat the grill to 180°C/350°F/Gas Mark 4.

2 Heat 1 tbsp of olive oil, cook 1 small chopped onion and 1 crushed garlic clove until soft.

3 Add 1 tsp each of ground cumin, ground coriander and ground turmeric and stir for 1 minute.

4 Add 115g/4 oz chopped mushrooms and cook until soft.

5 Remove the pan from the heat.

6 Cook, drain and rinse 400g/14 oz kidney beans (or use a can) and mash with fork (do not blend).

7 Stir the beans into the pan and form burger shapes with the mix.

8 Brush with oil and grill on the top shelf for 12 minutes.

9 Add some beef mince into the burger mix for meat eaters. Serve with salad or *Ratatouille (V) (page 44).*

Tip: *Make sure there is a bit of 'stick' when forming the burgers. If in doubt, add a little water to the mix.*

NOTES

Ratatouille (V)

Ingredients *Serves 4*

1 aubergine

1 courgette

2 onions

1 yellow or red pepper

3 garlic cloves

7 large tomatoes

handful fresh basil

1 tbsp olive oil

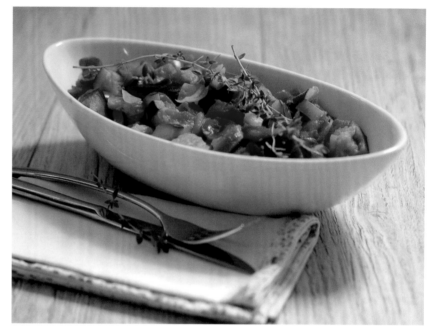

There are lots of veg in this. Make extra portions to freeze.

NOTES

1 Dice 1 aubergine and 1 courgette and place in a colander. Put to one side.

2 Dice 2 onions, 1 yellow or red pepper (de-seeded) and 7 large tomatoes (peeled).

3 In a large pan, fry the onions in 1 tbsp of olive oil with 3 crushed garlic cloves at medium heat until soft.

4 Add the aubergine, courgette, pepper and tomatoes. Add a handful of freshly chopped basil.

5 Bring to the boil stirring all the time. Reduce the heat, cover and simmer for about 40 minutes. Freeze any leftovers.

King Prawn Salad

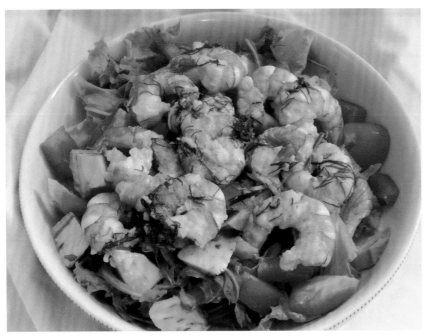

Ingredients *Serves 1*

generous glug of olive oil

2 large lettuce leaves

handful rocket

½ avocado

¼ red pepper

6 fresh or frozen king prawns

2 garlic cloves

2 tbsp lemon juice

fresh or dried dill

A good crunchy salad with meaty prawns! Love it!

1 Make a salad using 2 large lettuce leaves, a handful of rocket, ½ a chopped avocado and ¼ of a chopped red pepper.

2 Fry 6 fresh or frozen king prawns in a pan with a generous glug of olive oil and 2 chopped garlic cloves.

3 Add 2 tbsp of lemon juice, ground pepper and a handful of freshly chopped dill (dried dill would do).

4 Stir and take off the heat when the prawns are pink.

5 Add the cooked prawns to the salad.

6 Drizzle the remaining juice over the prawns and salad, then sprinkle with fresh dill if desired.

NOTES

Tasty Prawns

Ingredients *Serves 1*

1 garlic clove

1 tsp grated ginger

handful fresh coriander

½ tsp cumin seeds

sprinkle curry powder

handful fresh parsley

1 tbsp lemon juice

150g/5 oz pot natural yoghurt

8 fresh, uncooked king prawns, or 1 chicken breast if you prefer

olive or coconut oil

120g/4 oz of mung bean sprouts

NOTES

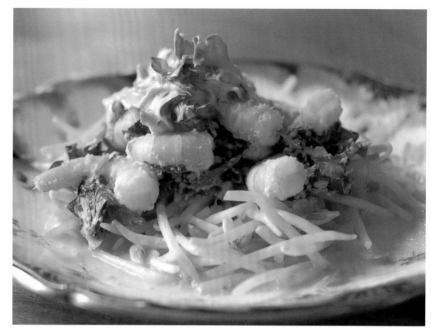

I love this dish for the zest and zing which is complimented nicely by the yoghurt.

1 For the sauce, mix together in a bowl 1 crushed garlic clove, 1 tsp of grated ginger, a handful of roughly chopped fresh coriander, ½ tsp of cumin seeds, a sprinkle of curry powder, a handful of parsley, 1 tbsp of lemon juice and a 150g/5 oz pot of natural yoghurt.

2 Put 2 tablespoons of the sauce to one side for serving.

3 Add 8 prawns to the sauce and mix well.

4 Gently fry the prawns in a glug of olive or coconut oil with the sauce until the flesh is pink.

5 Heat the sauce and prawns for a further 2 minutes. Serve on a bed of mung bean sprouts with the sauce you have set aside. *You can use chicken as an alternative.*

Salmon with Cucumber & Pomegranate Salad

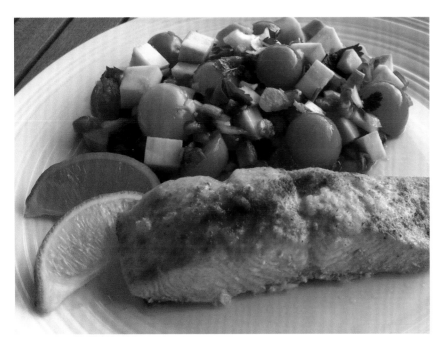

Ingredients *Serves 1*

1 salmon steak

olive oil

1 garlic clove

½ tsp paprika

½ cucumber

½ pomegranate

1 spring onion

handful cherry tomatoes

large handful fresh mint

2 limes

This is one of my favourites! Zany's genius salad had to feature in this book and it really works with the salmon. This is full of zesty flavours.

1 Preheat the oven to 180°C/350°F/Gas Mark 4.

2 Brush 1 salmon steak with olive oil on both sides, rub in 1 crushed garlic clove, a sprinkle of salt, pepper and ½ tsp of paprika.

3 Place on a baking tray on the middle shelf of the oven for 15 to 20 minutes. Don't let the salmon become too dry.

4 For the pomegranate salad, mix together ½ a peeled and diced cucumber, ½ a pomegranate (skin and pith removed), 1 finely chopped spring onion, a handful of chopped cherry tomatoes and a large handful of roughly chopped mint.

5 Add a couple of generous pinches of salt and then add the juice of 2 limes. Stir well.

6 Remove the salmon from the oven and serve with the pomegranate salad.

NOTES

Roasted Salmon with Pesto

Ingredients *Serves 1*

1 salmon fillet

½ lemon

½ red pepper

¼ courgette

1 to 2 tbsp flaked soya

Pesto Sauce (page 59)

mixed herbs

olive oil

To serve with Coriander and Cherry Tomatoes (after 28 day plan):

Ingredients

2 tbsp olive oil

8 cherry tomatoes

handful fresh coriander

2 tsp mirin

NOTES

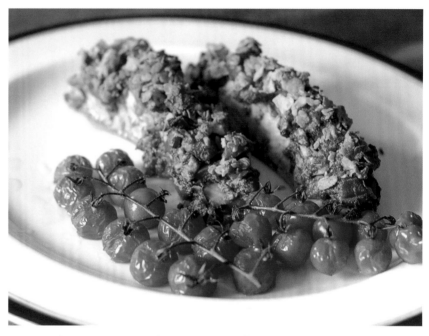

Serve with peas, or roasted tomatoes, or after the 28 day plan you can serve with Coriander and Cherry Tomatoes (V), see step 7.

1 Preheat the oven to 180°C/350°F/Gas Mark 4.

2 Place 1 salmon fillet on a baking tray.

3 Squeeze the lemon juice over the salmon and season with salt and pepper.

4 Make your own **Pesto Sauce (V)** (page 59). Any spare can be frozen (in individual portions) to use at another time.

5 Add ½ of a diced red pepper and ¼ of a small diced courgette to the pesto, to form a paste and spread over the fish.

6 Sprinkle 1 to 2 tbsp of flaked soya over the mix. Place the baking tray on the middle shelf for 20 minutes. Serve with peas or roast some cherry tomatoes in the oven, covered in olive oil and mixed herbs.

7 For **Coriander and Cherry Tomatoes** add 2 tbsp of olive oil and 2 tsp of mirin (after the 28 day plan) to 8 halved cherry tomatoes and stir. Chop up a handful of coriander and add to the tomatoes. Season with salt and pepper to taste. Try roasting the tomatoes in the oven as an alternative, before adding the other ingredients.

Smoked Salmon and Grapefruit

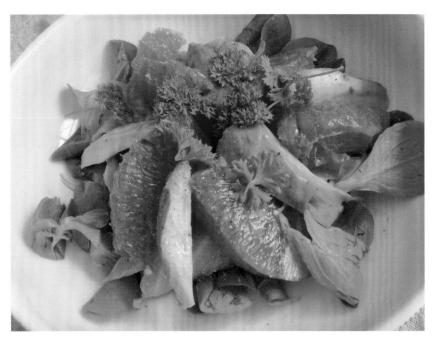

Ingredients *Serves 1*

½ grapefruit

1 avocado

1 tbsp olive oil

1 tsp balsamic vinegar

½ lemon

4 smoked salmon slices

handful lettuce leaves

parsley or coriander

My friend Natalie, (the most amazing lady I want to add), served this up one day. This has a quick and tasty sauce.

1 Skin ½ a grapefruit and 1 avocado and cut into segments.

2 To make the dressing, mix 1 tbsp of olive oil, 1 tsp of balsamic vinegar and ½ a lemon in a dish.

3 Coat 4 smoked salmon slices in the dressing and carefully do the same with the grapefruit and avocado segments.

4 Place a handful of lettuce leaves on a plate and then add the salmon slices, finishing with the grapefruit and avocado slices.

5 Pour the dressing over the top and garnish with parsley or coriander.

6 Add a dash of salt and pepper and serve.

Tip: Serve as a delicious quick starter.

NOTES

Baked Fish Fillet

Ingredients *Serves 1*

1 piece meaty white fish

2 garlic cloves

1 tbsp olive oil

1 tsp lemon juice

small handful fresh parsley and chives

pinch paprika

2 slices from large tomato

serve with steamed broccoli and/or Roasted Vegetables (p52)

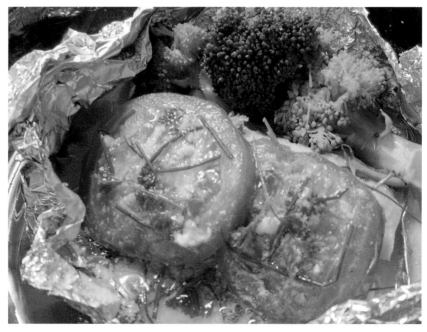

I love the unwrapping of the foil, like the unwrapping of a present …

NOTES

1 Preheat the oven to 200°C/400°F/Gas Mark 6.

2 Use a piece of meaty white fish (e.g. Cod). Line a baking tray with foil and combine 2 crushed cloves of garlic, 1 tbsp of olive oil and 1 tsp of lemon juice.

3 Add the fish and turn to coat both sides.

4 Sprinkle a small handful of chopped parsley and chives and a pinch of paprika, then cut 2 slices from a large tomato and lay them on top of the fish.

5 Finish by adding some salt and pepper and bake in the oven for about 15 minutes or just until the fish begins to flake. Serve with steamed broccoli and/or *Roasted Vegetables (V)* (page 52).

Fried Fish

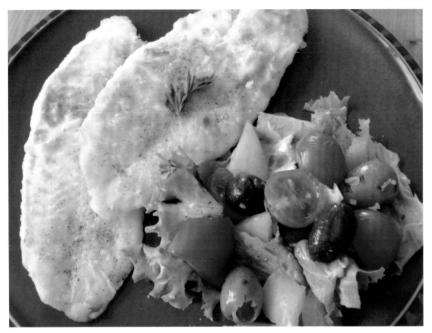

Ingredients *Serves 1*

1 or 2 pieces of white fish

1 tbsp of olive oil

(spelt flour)

salad garnish:

2 lettuce leaves

2 cherry tomatoes

4 olives

handful chopped yellow
and red peppers

My children love this; simple, tasty and easy!

1   Choose one or two pieces of white fish. Remove moisture by patting the fish with some kitchen towel.

2   Sprinkle salt on both sides of the fish and fry in 1 tbsp of olive oil. Serve with a salad garnish.

3   After Day 26, coat both sides of the fish with spelt flour and then add salt to the flour before frying the fish in olive oil. This will give the fish more texture.

NOTES

Roasted Vegetables (V)

Ingredients *Serves 1*

½ courgette

½ red pepper

1 onion

2 tbsp chopped herbs

1 tbsp olive oil

1 garlic clove

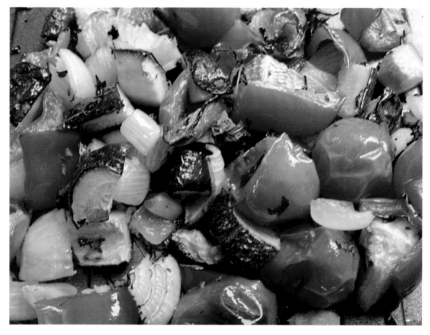

I love this for the taste and simplicity. Such a light dish. Great with a piece of fish.

NOTES

1 Preheat the oven to 220°C/425°F/Gas Mark 7.

2 Chop ½ a courgette, ½ a pepper and 1 onion and place in a roasting tin.

3 Add 2 tbsp of freshly chopped herbs of your choice, 1 tbsp of olive oil and 1 crushed garlic clove. Evenly spread the oil and garlic and turn the vegetables.

4 Bake in the oven for about 20 minutes, or until tender.

Fish Cakes

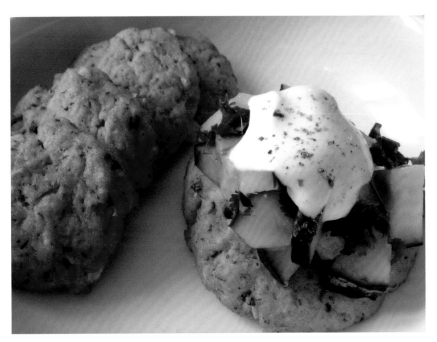

Ingredients *Serves 2*
150g/5 oz salmon meat
150g/5 oz crab meat
handful fresh coriander
½ spring onion
glug of olive oil

Cucumber Salsa
Ingredients
¼ cucumber
handful fresh coriander
½ lime
dollop of natural yoghurt
(½ red chilli)

It was quite tricky to work out a healthy fish cake recipe which tasted nice too. I am quite pleased with this one. I hope you enjoy it too.

1   Preheat the grill to 200°C/400°F/Gas Mark 6.

2   Blend 150g/5 oz salmon and 150g/5 oz crab meat with a handful of chopped coriander, ½ a chopped spring onion, a glug of olive oil, salt and ground pepper. Form fish cakes.

3   Cook on the top shelf until the fish cakes have browned slightly. Serve with **Cucumber Salsa.**

4   For the **Cucumber Salsa (V).** Mix in a bowl: ¼ of a cucumber (diced), a handful of chopped coriander, the juice of ½ a lime and some ground pepper. Add a dollop of natural yoghurt and if you want a kick, chop and add ½ a red chilli.

5   For a more meaty fish cake, break the salmon up with your hands and mix in the crab meat. Follow the rest of recipe and then fry them for 4 minutes on both sides on relatively high heat.

NOTES

DESSERT IDEAS
28 DAY PLAN

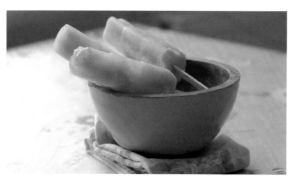

Lollies

Refreshing.

1 Use freshly squeezed fruit or pure juice. Pour into lolly moulds and freeze for a refreshing dessert.

Baked Pineapples

Serves 1. Yum!

1 Cut two rings (or 4 halves) from a pineapple (cored). Or use the whole pineapple cut into rings or halves. Dry on absorbent paper.

2 Sprinkle a little chilli powder and a generous amount of cinnamon over both sides of the pineapple. Use any fallen powder to coat the remaining pineapple. Grill on a high heat for 7 minutes on both sides, until slightly crispy.

3 After the 28 day plan, you can add 20g/1 oz of pure cane sugar to the mix. Cook each side on a high heat until brown.

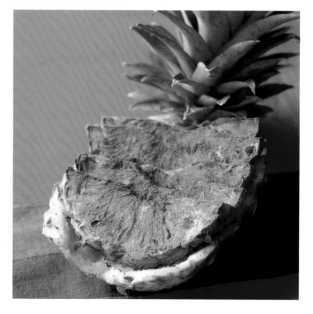

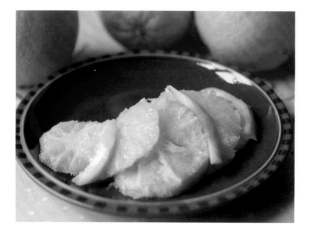

Stewed Orange

Serves 1. Good if you feel in need of a sweet fix.

1 Peel the skin of one orange and cut into slices.

2 Add 3 strips (5cm long) orange peel to a pan along with the orange slices and add 2 tbsp of water.

3 Cover the pan and stew for 10 minutes.

SAUCES AND TOPPINGS
28 DAY PLAN

If you have something in the fridge that needs jazzing up, try the following sauces or use some of the accompaniments suggested.

Lemon Dressing

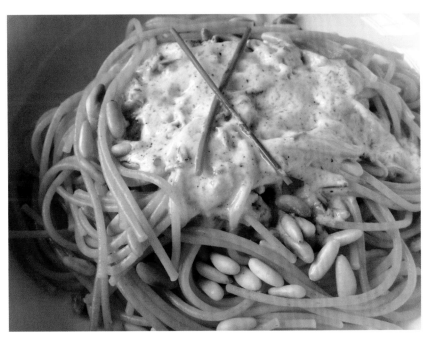

Ingredients *Serves 4.*

150g/5 oz natural yoghurt

1 tbsp olive oil

1 tbsp nut oil

2 tbsp lemon juice

¼ tsp grated lemon rind

2 tbsp fresh chives

NOTES

This is a really fresh tasting and versatile dressing. Good with pasta or fish.

Good with pasta or fish.

1 Mix 150g/5 oz natural yoghurt, 1 tbsp of olive oil, 1 tbsp of nut oil, 2 tbsp of lemon juice, a ¼ of a tsp of grated lemon rind, 2 tbsp of freshly chopped chives and a dash of salt and pepper.

2 To make a spaghetti dish: Cover the bottom of a saucepan with pine nuts and roast until brown.

3 Boil enough spaghetti for 4 people.

4 Place spaghetti in a bowl and top with pine nuts and then the lemon dressing. Serve with *Caramelized Onions: Moving Forward* (page 81).

Peanut Butter Sauce

Ingredients *Serves 4*

5 tbsp smooth peanut butter

2 tbsp soy sauce

1 tsp ground coriander

1 tsp ground cumin

1 lime

150ml/5 fl oz coconut milk

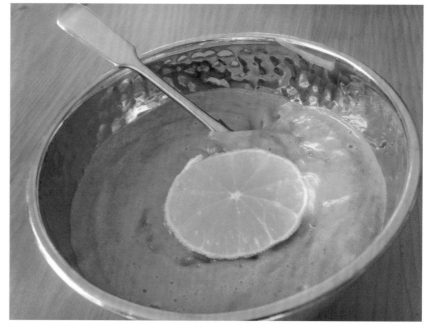

This is a good sauce to serve with a stir fry.

NOTES

1   With an electric mixer, blend together: 5 tbsp smooth peanut butter, 2 tbsp soy sauce, a dash of salt and pepper, 1 tsp ground coriander, 1 tsp ground cumin, juice of one lime and 150ml/5 fl oz coconut milk.

2   Heat for 2 minutes until slightly thickened and serve.

Herb Topping for Fish

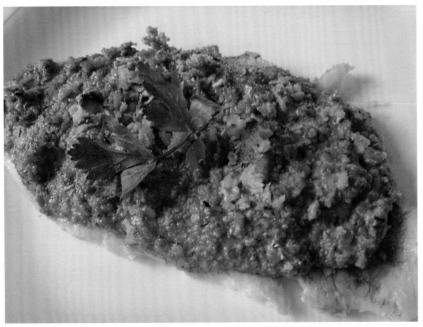

Ingredients *Serves 4*

2 tbsp nuts of your choice: walnut, cashew, brazil, almond

2 tbsp fresh dill

2 tbsp fresh parsley

2 tbsp fresh chives

6 plum tomatoes

200g/7 oz natural yoghurt

1 lemon

2 tbsp olive oil

8 tbsp flaked soya

This herb topping gives a nice crunchy taste to the fish and livens it up a bit.

1 In a blender, mix 2 tbsp of nuts of your choice (walnut, cashew, brazil, almond, etc).

2 Add 2 tbsp of freshly chopped dill, 2 tbsp of freshly chopped parsley, 2 tbsp of freshly chopped chives and 6 plum tomatoes and blend.

3 Add 200g/7 oz natural yoghurt, the juice of 1 lemon and 2 tbsp of olive oil and blend.

4 Mix in 8 tbsp of flaked soya with a fork.

5 Spread the topping on to the fish and sprinkle a dash of salt and generous amounts of flaked soya to finish. Bake in the oven until the fish is cooked.

6 Serve with *Honey-Glazed Carrots: Moving Forward* (page 82).

NOTES

Curry Yoghurt Sauce

Ingredients *Serves 4*

1 tsp curry powder

150g/5 oz pot natural yoghurt

handful fresh mint

2 tbsp olive oil

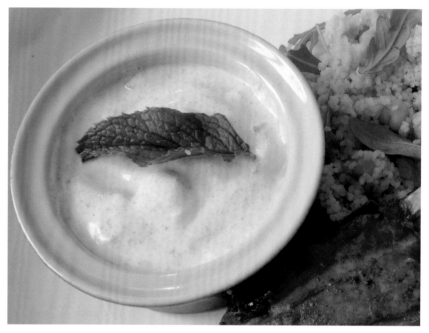

I use this sauce a lot to dress up a meat dish. It especially works well with lamb and chicken. Once again, it is so easy.

NOTES

1 Mix 1 tsp of curry powder and 2 tbsp of olive oil to 150g/5 oz pot of natural yoghurt and add a handful of freshly chopped mint.

2 Serve on top of meat. See the **Spicy Lamb with Warm Quinoa** recipe (page 71).

Pesto

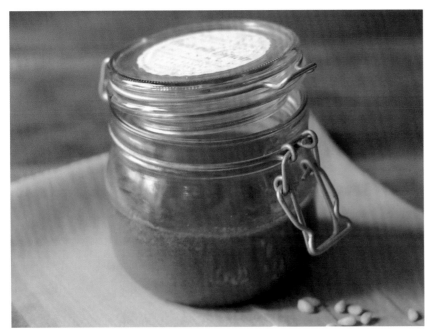

Ingredients *Serves 6-8*

125g/4 oz fresh basil

2 garlic cloves

100g/4 oz pine nuts

200ml/7 fl oz olive oil

It took me a while, but I think this pesto is just right! This is a real hit with my kids.

1 Blend 125g/4 oz basil leaves, 2 cloves of garlic, 100g/4 oz pine nuts, 200ml/7 fl oz olive oil, and a generous sprinkle of salt and pepper to taste.

NOTES

Simple Spinach Sauce

Ingredients *Serves 4*

200g/7 oz fresh spinach

1 tbsp natural veg stock powder

2 garlic cloves

olive oil

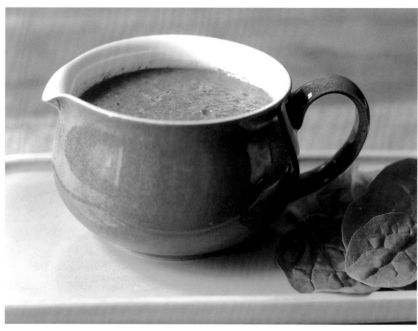

Does your meal look a little dry? If you have a bag of spinach, add a bit of stock and you have yourself a very quick sauce!

NOTES

1 Place 200g/7 oz fresh spinach in a pan with a glug of olive oil and 2 crushed garlic cloves.

2 When the spinach has reduced significantly in size, add 400ml/14 fl oz hot vegetable stock (using 1 tbsp of natural vegetable stock powder) and whizz in the blender et voilà – a swampy looking sauce with some flavour! Spinach sauce and pasta is a good combination.

SNACKS 28 DAY PLAN

*One of the best ways to stay on track during **Tidy the Temple** is to keep hunger pangs at bay. Preparing some snacks in advance will help you. Remember to eat every three hours and make sure you have a balance of protein and fruits/vegetables. Take a look at some of these ideas.*

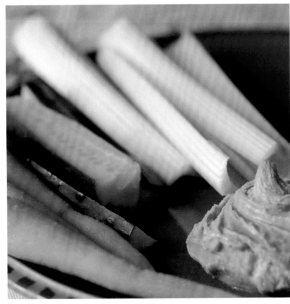

- Carrot/cucumber sticks and houmous or guacamole. Prepare a batch in advance. Keep in the fridge and, when you are going to work, make a snack box. See the recipes in the section *Tips on Having a Dinner Party* (page 101).
- Carrot sticks with pure peanut butter.
- Melon/grapefruit sprinkled with hemp seed and almonds.
- Fruit with a slice of chicken.
- Dry seaweed shredded on top of a slice of tempeh with a splash of soy sauce.
- Fruit and nuts.
- Slices of salmon and yoghurt with a sprinkle of paprika, wrapped in a lettuce leaf.
- Stewed Orange (page 54) with a handful of prawns.
- Prepare some slices of melon of your choice with 2 slices of parma ham.

NOTES

BREAKFAST IDEAS MOVING FORWARD

By now, you will have a good understanding of making healthy food choices. Including the recipes suggested for the 28 day plan, here are a few other recipes to help you move forward.

Peanut Banana Smoothie

Ingredients *Serves 1*

1 banana

3 tbsp natural yoghurt

125ml/4 fl oz rice milk

1 tbsp peanut butter

1 tsp runny honey

NOTES

This is smooth and creamy; fantastic with the peanut butter. This is for you Myles and Becs … you peanut butter lovers. Don't stay out in India too long.

1 Blend one banana, 3 tbsp of natural yoghurt, 125ml/4 fl oz rice milk, 1 tbsp of peanut butter and 1 tsp of runny honey and serve.

Summer Fruits Smoothie

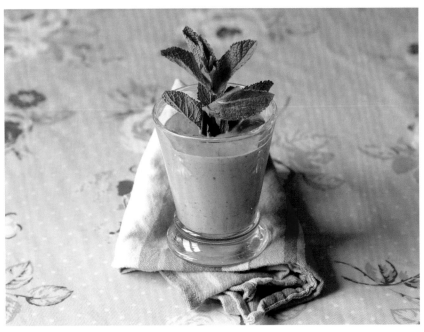

Ingredients *Serves 4*

1 old banana (frozen without the skin)

200g/7 oz frozen mixed fruits

200g/7 oz natural yoghurt

500ml/18 fl oz rice milk

honey to taste

Super fruity and easy. No fuss whatsoever.

Have you any old bananas that need using up? Then place them in the freezer (wrapped in foil without the skin) and use later to make tasty smoothies.

1 Unwrap the frozen banana from the foil, and blend with the 200g/7 oz frozen mixed fruits, 200g/7 oz natural yoghurt and 500ml/18 fl oz rice milk.

2 Add honey to taste and serve.

NOTES

Mini Frittatas

Ingredients

Makes 15 frittatas

olive oil

⅓ courgette

⅓ red pepper

4 eggs

150ml/5 fl oz rice milk

1 tbsp freshly chopped thyme

150g/5 oz goat's cheese

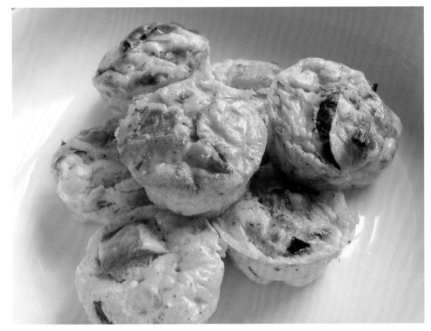

I love these as they look so cute and taste so good.

NOTES

1 Preheat the oven to 190°C/375°F/Gas Mark 5.

2 Line a muffin tray with olive oil.

3 Finely chop ⅓ of a courgette and ⅓ of a pepper and soften in the oven.

4 In a bowl, mix together 4 eggs, 150ml/5 fl oz rice milk, ½ tsp of salt, ½ tsp of pepper and 1 tbsp of freshly chopped thyme.

5 Add the courgette and the pepper.

6 Add 150g/5 oz goat's cheese (chopped in small pieces).

7 Spoon the mixture into the muffin cases, ensuring the cases have a cheese and veg mix.

8 Bake for 15 minutes and serve warm.

Pineapple and Carrot Muffins

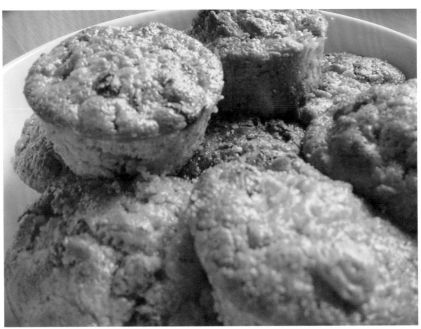

Ingredients

Makes 12 muffins

200g/7 oz spelt flour

2 tsp baking powder

2 tsp cinnamon

50ml/2 fl oz grape seed oil

50ml/2 fl oz rice milk

90g/3 oz pure cane sugar

2 eggs

120g/4 oz carrots

225g/8 oz crushed pineapple

My lovely friend Sarah made these for me one day. I just had to include them in here. These have a different twist but taste just as good.

1 Preheat the oven to 180°C/350°F/Gas Mark 4.

2 In a bowl, sift 200g/7 oz spelt flour, 2 tsp of baking powder, 2 tsp of cinnamon and ½ tsp of salt. Mix well.

3 Beat 50ml/2 fl oz grape seed oil, 50ml/2 fl oz rice milk, 90g/3 oz pure cane sugar and 2 eggs until well blended.

4 Add 120g/4 oz finely grated carrots and 225g/8 oz crushed pineapple.

5 Pour the batter into the oiled muffin tray and bake for 40 minutes. Leave to cool completely in the tray before serving.

NOTES

Honey Drenched Nuts

Ingredients

nuts of your choice:
unsalted cashew, walnut,
whole almonds, brazil,
pecan, macadamia,
sunflower

clear honey

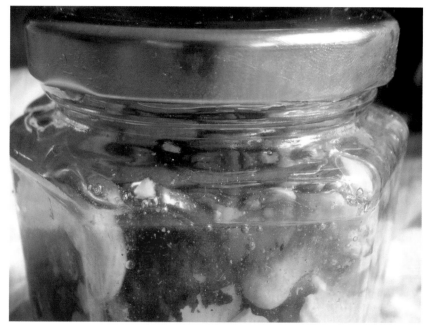

This is easy to make and doubles up as a nice little present too!

NOTES

1 Place nuts of your choice in a glass jar (unsalted cashew, walnut, whole almonds, brazil, pecan, macadamia, sunflower).

2 Fill the jar with clear honey until all the nuts are coated.

3 Place the lid on the jar. Use on yoghurt or salads.

Oat Surprise

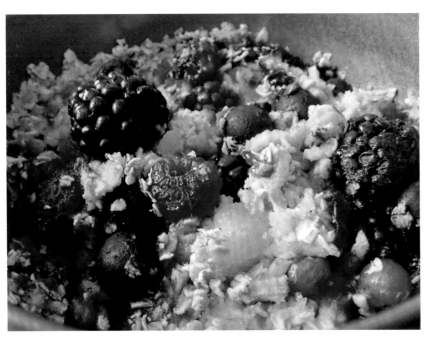

Ingredients *Serves 1*

¼ apple

2 tbsp apple compote

20g/1 oz oats

handful frozen mixed berries

The health benefits of oats should not be sniffed at. This whole grain has been linked to increasing appetite control hormones, reducing blood pressure, increasing immune defenses and so much more. Start the day off with 'Oat Surprise'.

1 Preheat the oven to 180°C/350°F/Gas Mark 4.

2 In a bowl, add 20g/1 oz oats, ¼ of a grated apple, 2 tbsp of apple compote, 2 tbsp of water, a handful of frozen mixed berries and mix carefully.

3 Cook for 20 minutes.

> **Tip:** *Make a few batches and freeze. After defrosting, add some apple juice and compote.*

NOTES

LUNCH AND DINNER IDEAS MOVING FORWARD

Coconut Millet Salad (V)

Ingredients *Serves 4*

250g/9 oz millet

1 tbsp natural vegetable stock powder

175g/6 oz ready to eat soft dried apricots

small bunch fresh chives

2 tbsp unsweetened desiccated coconut

½ tsp cinnamon

Dressing

1 tbsp olive oil

juice of ½ orange

½ tsp finely grated orange rind

1 tsp wholegrain mustard

1 tsp honey

2 tbsp fresh mint

NOTES

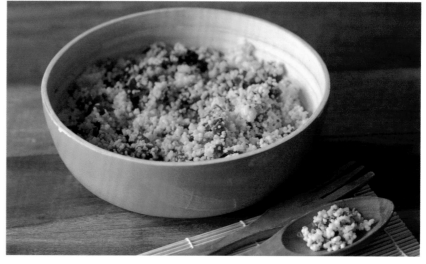

A refreshing side dish.

1 Drain and rinse the millet under warm water.

2 Cook 250g/9 oz millet according to the instructions on the packet. Transfer to a serving bowl.

3 Add 1 tbsp of natural vegetable stock powder to 100ml/4 fl oz boiling water. Stir well and pour evenly over the millet.

4 Slice 175g/6 oz ready to eat soft dried apricots thinly and add to the millet.

5 Snip a small bunch of chives over the apricots.

6 When the millet is cool, mix 2 tbsp of unsweetened desiccated coconut, ½ tsp of cinnamon and season to taste.

7 *Dressing:* Mix 1 tbsp of olive oil and the juice of half an orange with ½ tsp finely grated orange rind in a small bowl. Add 1 tsp of wholegrain mustard and 1 tsp of clear honey. Mix and pour over the millet and leave to chill for 1 hour to allow the flavour to develop. Serve with 2 tbsp of chopped mint leaves.

Vegetable Stir Fry (V)

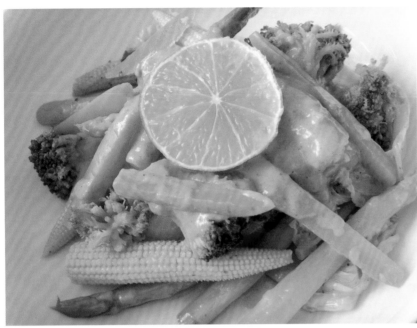

A flavoursome stir fry. If you have time, make the Peanut Butter Sauce. It compliments the dish nicely.

Ingredients *Serves 4*

3 tbsp nut oil

3 tbsp sesame oil

3 garlic cloves

2.5cm/1 inch fresh ginger

3 carrots

350g/12 oz broccoli florets

250g/9 oz asparagus tips

2 large spring onions

4 baby corn

300g/11 oz Chinese leaf

4 tbsp soy sauce

3 tbsp mirin

1 tbsp sesame seeds

add Peanut Butter sauce (page 56) if desired

NOTES

1 Place a frying pan or wok over high heat.

2 Add 3 tbsp of nut oil, 3 tbsp of sesame oil and 3 chopped garlic cloves and heat for 2 minutes.

3 Add these ingredients to the pan: 2.5cm/1 inch chopped fresh ginger, 3 finely chopped carrots, 350g/12 oz broccoli florets, 250g/9 oz asparagus tips, 2 large chopped spring onions (cut diagonally) and 4 baby corn.

4 Cover the pan and cook for 8 minutes. Stir occasionally.

5 Add 300g/11 oz sliced Chinese leaf.

6 Add 4 tbsp of soy sauce and 3 tbsp of mirin.

7 Cook for another 3 minutes. Take off heat and sprinkle over 1 tbsp of sesame seeds.

8 Add Peanut Butter Sauce (page 56) if desired.

Chicken and Rice

Ingredients *Serves 4*

500g/17.5 oz wild or brown rice

olive oil

4 chicken thighs

2 onions

2 garlic cloves

1 tbsp tomato purée

1 tsp paprika

1 tbsp natural chicken stock powder

1 tbsp wholegrain mustard

dollop natural yoghurt

1 yellow pepper

1 red pepper

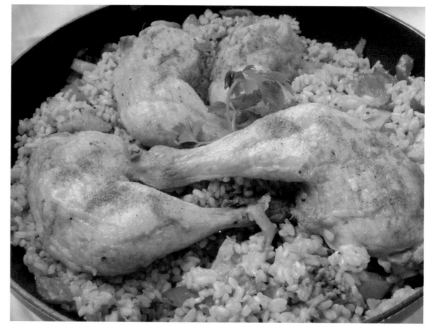

A really hearty dish. Make in advance and freeze.

NOTES

1 Using a rice cooker or a pan, cook 500g/17.5 oz of wild or brown rice (rinsed), enough for 4 people.

2 Place 4 chicken thighs on a baking tray. Cover both sides with olive oil and season with salt and pepper. Cook in the oven until browned.

3 Heat 2 tbsp of olive oil in the pan and add 2 diced onions, 1 diced yellow pepper, 1 diced red pepper and add 2 crushed garlic cloves. Cook for a few minutes.

4 Add the rice and 1 tbsp of tomato purée and cook for 1 minute.

5 Stir in 1 tsp of paprika, 1 tbsp of wholegrain mustard and 300ml/ 11 fl oz hot chicken stock (using 1 tbsp of natural chicken stock powder).

6 Bring to the boil and allow the liquid to reduce for 2 minutes.

7 Return the chicken to the pan. Reduce heat, cover and simmer for 10 minutes or until liquid has reduced.

8 Stir well and simmer uncovered until the mixture has thickened.

9 Serve with a dollop of natural yoghurt.

Spicy Lamb with Warm Quinoa

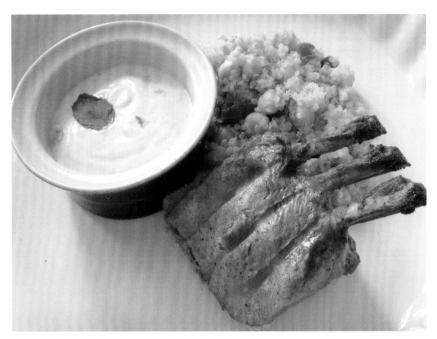

Ingredients *Serves 4*

250g/9 oz quinoa

handful rocket

zest 1 lemon

1 tbsp natural chicken stock powder

1 tsp mild chilli powder

3 tsp curry powder

olive oil

500g/17 oz pot natural yoghurt

rack of lamb (600g/21 oz)

handful fresh mint

400g/14 oz chickpeas or a can

A favourite meal to serve to guests – quick, simple and so tasty! The lamb and dressing work a treat; the quinoa adds a lovely taste and texture.

1 Heat the grill to medium.

2 Rinse 250g/9 oz quinoa under warm water. Cook the quinoa according to the instructions on the packet. Transfer to a serving bowl.

3 Add 400g/14 oz rinsed and cooked chickpeas (or a can) and the zest of 1 lemon. Add 1 tbsp of natural chicken stock powder to 100ml/4 fl oz boiling water. Stir well and pour evenly over the quinoa and chickpeas.

4 In a bowl, mix together 1 tsp of mild chilli powder, 2 tsp of curry powder, ½ tsp of salt and a sprinkle of pepper, a glug of olive oil and 4 tbsp of natural yoghurt.

5 Smear the paste over the rack of lamb, season to taste, then grill for 3 to 4 minutes on each side until crisp outside and cooked in the middle. Cover, then set aside for a few minutes.

6 In a small jug, mix 1 tsp of curry powder into 150g/5 oz pot of natural yoghurt and add a handful of chopped mint. Use as a dressing for the lamb. Fold a handful of rocket through the warm quinoa. Serve with the chops and dressing.

NOTES

Beef Curry with Pumpkin and Prunes

Ingredients *Serves 4 to 6*

2 large onions

2 garlic cloves

2 tsp ground cumin

2 tsp curry powder

800g/28 oz stewing beef

4 ripe tomatoes

600g/21 oz pumpkin

2 tbsp natural beef stock powder

2 bay leaves

3 handfuls pitted prunes

3 tbsp ground almonds

500g/18 oz pot natural yoghurt

brown rice

glug olive oil

handful fresh coriander

NOTES

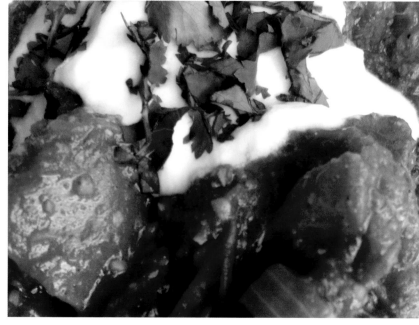

The prunes are a fantastic addition.

1   Preheat the oven to 170C°/340°F/Gas Mark 4.

2   On the hob, heat a good glug of olive oil in a large pan. Gently fry 2 large chopped onions and 2 finely chopped garlic cloves. Add 2 tsp of ground cumin and 2 tsp of curry powder and fry for a minute or two.

3   Add 800g/28 oz (stewing) beef and coat the beef in the mixture turning regularly until browned. Add 4 ripe chopped tomatoes and bring to the simmer.

4   Add 600g/21 oz pumpkin (skinned and cut into chunks). Add 400ml/14 fl oz hot beef stock (using 2 tbsp of natural beef stock powder), 2 bay leaves, 1 tsp of salt and a sprinkle of pepper.

5   Simmer, then add 3 handfuls of prunes and 3 tbsp of ground almonds.

6   Transfer to a dish, cook in the oven for an hour until the beef is tender.

7   Serve with a generous amount of chopped coriander and mix in 500g/17 oz natural yoghurt. Serve on a bed of brown rice, season to taste.

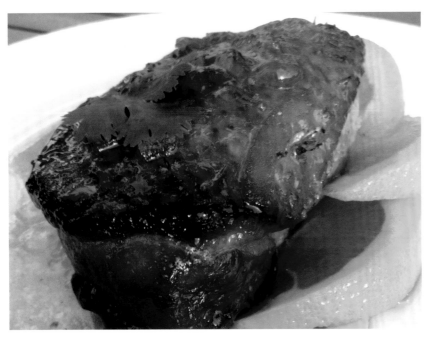

BBQ Orange Duck

Ingredients *Serves 4*

370g/13 oz marmalade
(100% fruit spread)

4 duck breasts

4 tbsp runny honey

serve with Courgette and
Almonds (page 39) and/or
Coconut Millet Salad
(page 68)

This turns out so well when barbecued but fine if you want to cook it in an oven. Choose this for a quick and impressive meal.

You can marinade this the night before.

NOTES

1 In a shallow dish, mix 370g/13 oz marmalade (100% fruit spread) and 4 tbsp of clear runny honey. Season with salt and pepper.

2 Reserve ⅓ of the marinade and set aside.

3 Place 4 duck breasts in the marinade, cover and place in the fridge overnight. Alternatively, if you have run out of time, marinate for 2 hours in the fridge.

4 Barbecue the duck until tender and pour the reserved marinade over the cooked duck.

5 Alternatively you can cook the duck in the oven at 200°C/400°F/Gas Mark 6 until tender. Put any left over marinade in a jug so that people can help themselves to more.

6 Serve with *Courgette and Almonds (V)* (page 39) and/or *Coconut Millet Salad (V) (page 68).*

Spaghetti Bolognese

Ingredients *Serves 4*

2 tsp olive oil

2 garlic cloves

1 onion

1 carrot

500g/18 oz beef mince

200g/7 oz mushrooms

2 tsp Italian herbs

1 tsp oregano

3 good sized tomatoes (or 400g can)

2 tbsp tomato purée

2 tsp Worcestershire sauce

handful fresh basil leaves

50ml/2 fl oz rice milk

wholewheat or spelt pasta

NOTES

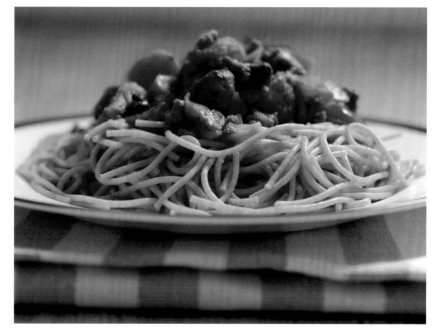

There are so many good bologneses out there but this is a firm favourite with the children.

1 Heat 2 tsp of olive oil in a large saucepan.

2 Add 2 crushed garlic cloves, 1 chopped onion and 1 chopped carrot. Stir until onions have softened.

3 Add 500g/18 oz beef mince and cook until meat is browned. Then add 200g/7 oz mushrooms, 2 tsp of Italian herbs and 1 tsp of oregano and cook for a further 2 minutes.

4 Add 3 chopped tomatoes (or a 400g can) and add 1 tsp of salt, a sprinkle of pepper, 2 tbsp of tomato purée, 2 tsp of Worcestershire sauce and a handful of chopped basil leaves. Simmer for 25 minutes.

5 Pour 50ml/2 fl oz rice milk and stir well. Cover the pan and simmer for a further 10 minutes, stirring occasionally.

6 Boil some wholewheat or spelt pasta according to instructions on the packet and serve with bolognese and a handful of chopped basil leaves.

7 For a *Vegetarian Bolognese (V)*, leave out the meat and use slices of tempeh (2 x 200g/7 oz pack). Leave out the Worcestershire sauce.

Meaty Fish with Japanese Sauce

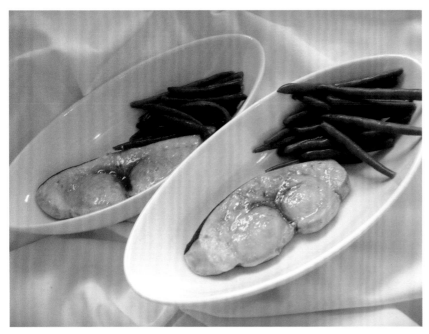

Ingredients *Serves 2*

2 pieces of swordfish

1 lemon

olive oil

1 tbsp pure cane sugar

1 tbsp mirin or fish sauce

1 tbsp soy sauce

serve with a handful of beans or broccoli or Raw Broccoli Salad (page 76)

My mum often uses this sauce in a variety of Japanese dishes. It brings out the flavour in the fish nicely.

1 Choose 2 pieces of fish (e.g. swordfish).

2 Season with the juice of 1 lemon and olive oil and bake in the oven until cooked.

3 Mix 50ml/2 fl oz hot water in a pot with 1 tbsp of mirin (or fish sauce), 1 tbsp of pure cane sugar and 1 tbsp of soy sauce. The combination between sweet and sour is delicious.

4 Pour over the fish when cooked and serve with steamed vegetables. Beans or broccoli are a good choice or serve with *Raw Broccoli Salad* (page 76).

5 Use any leftover sauce as gravy for the vegetables.

NOTES

Raw Broccoli Salad (V)

Ingredients *Serves 4*

100g/4 oz flaked almonds

500g/18 oz natural yoghurt

500g/18 oz broccoli florets

160g/6 oz raisins

40g/1 oz sultanas

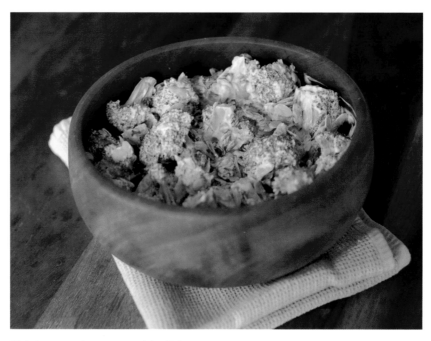

This is a great summer side dish.

NOTES

1 Toast 100g/4 oz flaked almonds until brown.

2 Mix 500g/18 oz natural yoghurt, ½ tsp of pepper and ½ tsp of salt.

3 Add 500g/18 oz raw broccoli florets and mix well.

4 Add 160g/6 oz raisins and 40g/1 oz sultanas and the toasted almonds.

5 Transfer to a serving dish.

Sardine Pasta

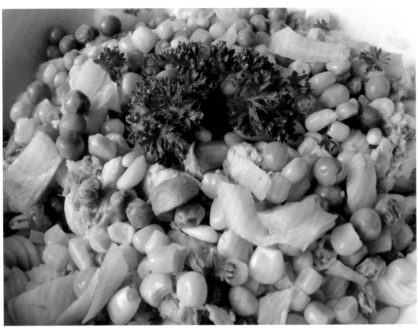

Ingredients *Serves 4*

200g/7 oz wholewheat or spelt pasta

½ fennel

2 tbsp olive oil

100g/4 oz frozen peas

125g/4 oz frozen sweetcorn

125g/4 oz tin sardines

4 chopped anchovies

handful capers

2 handfuls pine nuts

handful fresh parsley

This has a bit of a fishy kick– a great hit with my children.

1 Boil 200g/7 oz wholewheat or spelt pasta.

2 In a steamer, place ½ a fennel (diced) and add to a pan with 100g/4 oz frozen peas and 125g/4 oz frozen sweetcorn. Steam until soft.

3 Drain the pasta and coat with 2 tbsp of olive oil.

4 Spread the following evenly over the pasta: 125g/4 oz tin chopped sardines, 4 chopped anchovies, a handful of capers and 2 handfuls of pine nuts.

5 Finish by adding the cooked fennel, peas and sweetcorn. Garnish with a handful of chopped parsley.

NOTES

Oriental Grilled Tuna Steaks

Ingredients *Serves 2*

2 tuna steaks

1 spring onion

25ml/1 fl oz mirin

25ml/1 fl oz soy sauce

6 tbsp coconut or olive oil

1 tbsp grated ginger

handful dry or fresh seaweed

serve with brown rice, green beans or Soy Mung Bean Sprouts (page 27)

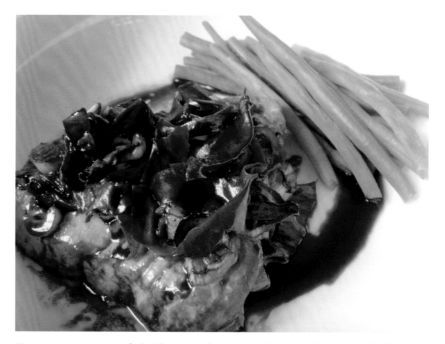

Time your tuna carefully if you prefer them a little on the rare side. The seaweed adds a bit of colour and nutrition!

NOTES

1   Place 2 tuna steaks in a shallow baking tray.

2   In a bowl, combine 1 chopped spring onion, 25ml/1 fl oz mirin, 25ml/1 fl oz soy sauce, 6 tbsp of coconut or olive oil, 1 tbsp of grated ginger and 1 tsp of ground pepper.

3   Cover and marinate in the fridge for 2 hours.

4   Preheat the grill to a high heat.

5   Cook the steaks for two minutes per side for a rare tuna steak. If you prefer your steak more cooked, simply leave it grilling for longer. Heat the remaining marinade in a pan.

6   Spoon the marinade over the tuna steaks. Add some dry or fresh seaweed.

7   Serve with brown rice, green beans or *Soy Mung Bean Sprouts (V)* (page 27).

Creamy Pumpkin Soup (V)

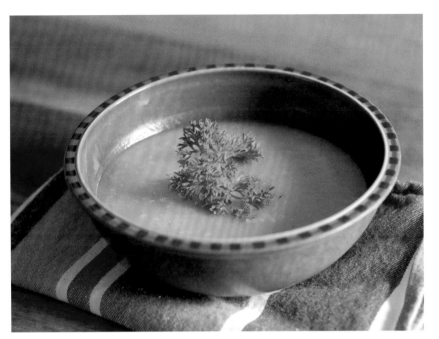

Ingredients *Serves 4*

1kg/2.2lbs pumpkin

1 onion

2 tbsp olive oil

½ tsp nutmeg

½ tsp pure cane sugar

2 tbsp natural veg stock powder

The nutmeg really adds a great flavour to the pumpkin soup. Feel free to add some more as preferred.

1   Remove the skin from 1kg/2.2lbs pumpkin, and de-seed then dice.

2   Fry 1 chopped onion in 2 tbsp of olive oil until soft.

3   Add the pumpkin chunks, 1 tsp of salt, ½ tsp of nutmeg and ½ tsp of pure cane sugar.

4   Stir well and then add 900ml/32 fl oz hot vegetable stock (using 2 tbsp of natural vegetable stock powder).

5   Stir, cover and simmer for 25 minutes. Blend, season to taste and serve.

NOTES

Quick Salad Dressing (V)

Ingredients

glug of olive oil

mirin (or clear honey)

soy sauce

mixed herbs to taste

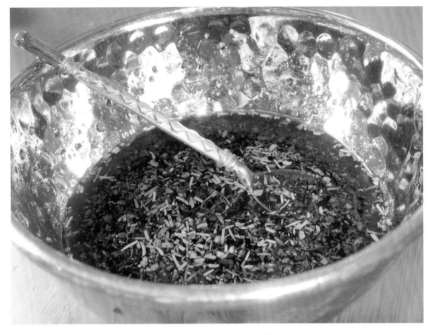

This is a really quick dressing which can be added to any salad. Experiment with different dried and fresh herbs.

NOTES

1   Mix together a glug of olive oil, mirin, soy sauce and mixed herbs to taste. Clear honey can be used as a substitute for mirin.

Caramelized Onions (V)

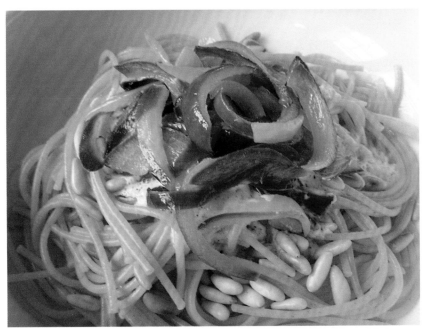

Ingredients *Serves 4*

1 tbsp olive oil

2 medium red onions

2 medium white onions

1 tbsp pure cane sugar

This is a great addition to pasta or as a side serving. The sweetness of the onions provides a good contrast to something savoury.

1 Heat 1 tbsp of olive oil in a pan.

2 Add 2 chopped medium red onions and 2 medium white onions to the pan and heat for 3 to 4 minutes.

3 Add 1 tbsp of pure cane sugar and raise the heat for 2 to 3 minutes, stirring until the onions are shiny.

NOTES

Honey-Glazed Carrots (V)

Ingredients *Serves 4*

450g/16 oz carrots

1 garlic clove

2 tbsp fresh rosemary

1 tbsp nut oil

2 tbsp olive oil

2 tbsp clear honey

1 tbsp lemon juice

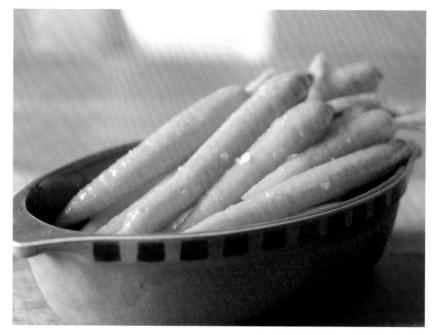

The lemon and rosemary work well in this dish.

NOTES

1 In a medium saucepan, bring some water to the boil and add a dash of salt.

2 Cook 450g/16 oz carrots until tender.

3 Drain the carrots and in a frying pan, add 1 crushed garlic clove, 2 tbsp of freshly chopped rosemary leaves, 1 tbsp of nut oil, 2 tbsp of olive oil and cook until the garlic is golden brown.

4 Add 2 tbsp of clear honey and 1 tbsp of lemon juice, and make sure the carrots are coated in the honey glaze. Add a dash of salt and serve immediately with the rest of the honey glaze from the pan.

DESSERT IDEAS MOVING FORWARD

To reduce your sugar intake but still enjoy sweet treats, try the recipes using organic, pure cane sugar and simply reduce the amount of sugar suggested, or use organic, unprocessed honey, or organic puréed fruit.

Blueberry and Cinnamon Cake

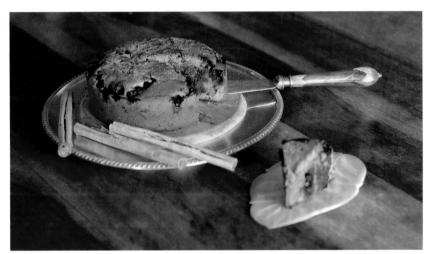

This is one of my favourites.

Ingredients *Serves 6*

olive oil for lining the tray plus 4 tbsp

4 tbsp nut oil

140g/5 oz pure cane sugar

140g/5 oz ground almonds

140g/5 oz buckwheat flour

3 eggs

1 tsp ground cinnamon plus for dusting

2 tsp vanilla extract

225g/8 oz blueberries

1 Preheat the oven to 180°C/350°F/Gas Mark 4.

2 Grease a 17cm to 19cm round cake tin with olive oil. (Do not use a larger tin.)

3 Put 4 tbsp of nut oil, 4 tbsp of olive oil, 140g/5 oz pure cane sugar, 140g/5 oz ground almonds, 140g/5 oz buckwheat flour, 3 eggs, 1 tsp ground cinnamon and 2 tsp of vanilla extract into a bowl and beat well with an electric mixer.

4 Spread ¾ of the mixture into the prepared tin and flatten lightly using the back of a fork.

5 Sprinkle over 225g/8 oz blueberries and dot over the remaining cake mixture so that it covers the fruit.

6 Place the tin on a baking sheet and bake for approximately 1-1¼ hours and check it is cooked through. Leave to cool in the tin.

7 Sift a little ground cinnamon over the top of the cake and serve.

NOTES

Grape Cake

Ingredients *Serves 6 to 8*

450g/16 oz seedless black grapes

225g/8 oz spelt flour plus for dusting grapes

140g/5 oz pure cane sugar

1 tsp baking powder

5 eggs

2 tbsp grape seed oil plus for lining the tray

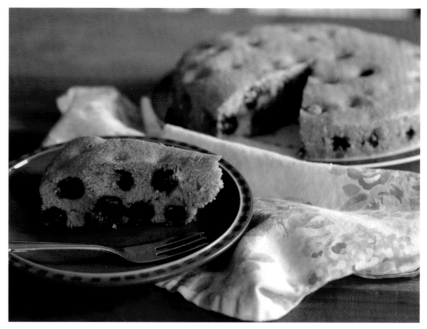

The grapes give a lovely sweetness to this cake.

NOTES

1   Preheat the oven to 180°C/350°F/Gas Mark 4.

2   Grease a round 21cm cake tin with grape seed oil.

3   Dust 450g/16 oz seedless black grapes with a little spelt flour.

4   Put 225g/8 oz spelt flour, 140g/5 oz pure cane sugar and 1 tsp of baking powder into a large bowl.

5   Add 5 eggs, one at a time, beating well with a wooden spoon after each addition, until there is a batter.

6   Add the grapes and 2 tbsp of grape seed oil and mix together.

7   Pour the mixture into the tin and bake for approximately 30 to 40 minutes on the middle shelf, until golden. Turn out and cool on a wire rack.

Lemon Drizzle

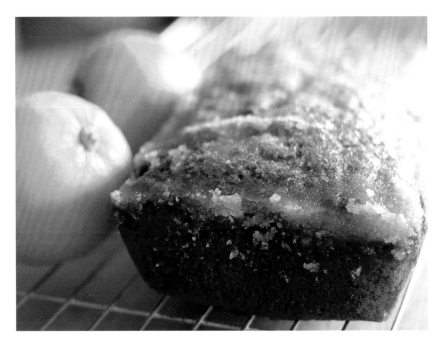

Ingredients *Serves 6 to 8*

4 tbsp grape seed oil

310g/11 oz pure cane sugar

4 eggs

140g/5 oz spelt flour

2 lemons

No one can resist a bit of Lemon Drizzle. I am afraid this cake doesn't last very long.

1   Preheat the oven to 180°C/356°F/Gas Mark 4.

2   In a bowl, mix 4 tbsp of grape seed oil and 225g/8 oz pure cane sugar.

3   Mix in 4 eggs.

4   Sift 140g/5 oz spelt flour and then add the zest of 1 lemon.

5   Spoon the mixture into a lined loaf tin.

6   Bake for 40 to 50 minutes on the middle shelf.

7   While the cake is cooling in the tin, mix the juice of 2 lemons with 85g/3 oz pure cane sugar.

8   Prick the warm cake all over with a skewer and then pour over the drizzle. The juice will sink and the sugar will form a crisp topping.

9   Leave in the tin until completely cool.

NOTES

Honey Cake

Ingredients *Serves 6 to 8*

175g/6 oz clear honey plus 1 tbsp

3 tbsp olive oil

2 tsp baking powder

95g/3 oz pure cane sugar

2 eggs

200g/7 oz oat flour (or put oats in a blender to make your oat flour)

50ml/2 fl oz grape seed oil plus for lining the tray

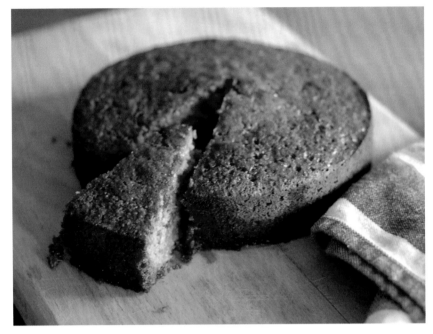

This cake is a must for honey-lovers.

NOTES

1   Preheat the oven to 180°C/350°F/Gas Mark 4.

2   Line the bottom of an 18cm/7in tin with grape seed oil.

3   Measure 175g/6 oz clear honey, 3 tbsp of olive oil and 95g/3 oz pure cane sugar into a large pan.

4   Add 1 tbsp of water and heat on low until mixed and melted.

5   Remove from the heat and wait until the pan has cooled a little before adding 2 beaten eggs, 2 tsp of baking powder and 200g/7 oz oat flour.

6   Spoon the mixture into the cake tin and bake for 50 minutes until the sponge is soft to touch and shrinking slightly from the sides of the tin.

7   Cool slightly in the tin before turning on to a wire rack.

8   While the cake is warm, make the honey icing by mixing 50ml/2 fl oz grape seed oil and 1 tbsp of honey with 2 to 3 tsp of hot water.

9   Put the cake on a plate and trickle the honey icing over the cake. Leave until the honey has soaked into the sponge.

Avocado Bread Cake

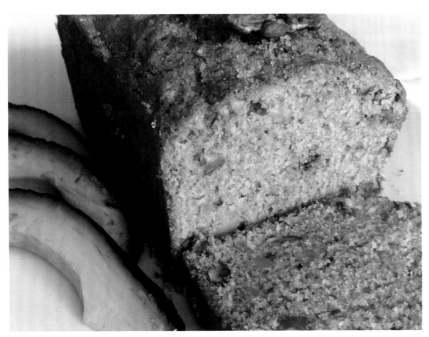

This is a great bread cake for afternoon tea.

Ingredients *Serves 8*

50ml/2 fl oz grape seed oil

200g/7 oz pure cane sugar plus 25g/1 oz sugar for topping

2 eggs

2 bananas

1 avocado

2 handfuls pecan nuts (plus 5 for decoration)

300g/10 oz spelt flour

2 tsp baking powder

rice milk in reserve

1   Preheat the oven to 180°C/350°F/Gas Mark 4.

2   Grease the sides of a loaf tin and line the base with greaseproof paper.

3   Mix 50ml/2 fl oz grape seed oil, 200g/7 oz pure cane sugar, 2 beaten eggs, 2 mashed bananas, a finely chopped avocado and 2 handfuls of chopped pecan nuts.

4   Add 300g/10 oz spelt flour with 2 tsp of baking powder and stir well.

5   Add some rice milk if the mixture is not sticky in consistency. Pour the mix into the loaf tin and then place 5 whole pecan nuts decoratively in a line, on top of the cake. Cook for about 45 minutes on the middle shelf.

6   Sprinkle 25g/1 oz of pure cane sugar over the top of the loaf after cooked. Let it cool and then serve.

NOTES

Oat Spice Cake

Ingredients *Serves 9 to 12*

85g/3 oz oats

1 tbsp nut oil

200g/7 oz pure cane sugar plus 4 tbsp for topping

3 eggs

100g/4 oz spelt flour

½ tsp baking powder

2 tbsp ground cinnamon, plus 2 tsp for topping

1 tsp ground nutmeg

grape seed oil for lining tray

½ tsp vanilla extract

40g/1 oz pecan nuts

sprinkle unsweetened desiccated coconut

NOTES

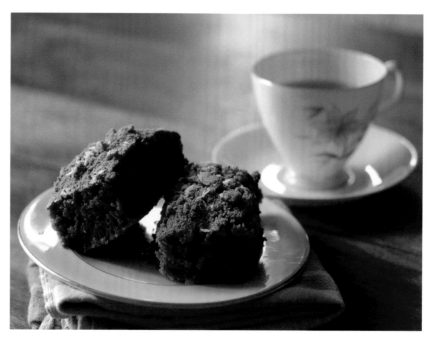

The smell of this cake reminds me of Christmas. This is a mélange of textures and tastes!

1 Preheat the oven to 180°C/350°F/Gas Mark 4.

2 In a bowl, pour 240ml/8 fl oz boiling water over 85g/3 oz oats.

3 Add 1 tbsp of nut oil, cover and let stand for 15 minutes.

4 In another bowl, stir in 200g/7 oz pure cane sugar, 3 eggs, 100g/4 oz spelt flour, ½ tsp of baking powder, 2 tbsp of ground cinnamon and 1 tsp of ground nutmeg. Add to the oats.

5 Bake in a 18/19cm rectangular tin, lined with grape seed oil, for 35 minutes.

6 Meanwhile for the topping, mix ½ tsp of vanilla extract, 2 tsp of ground cinnamon, 4 tbsp of pure cane sugar and 40g/1 oz finely chopped pecan nuts. Spread over the cake once cooked and while hot.

7 Finish by sprinkling unsweetened desiccated coconut over the top.

Oat Biscuits

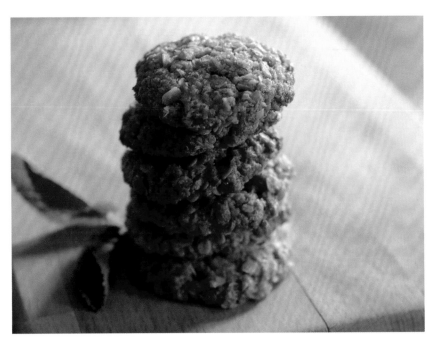

Ingredients

Makes approx 10-12

4 tbsp olive oil

4 tbsp nut oil

4 tbsp clear honey (plus 1 to 2 in reserve)

115g/4 oz pure cane sugar

85g/3 oz oats (or put oats in a blender to make your oat flour)

55g/2 oz unsweetened desiccated coconut

115g/4 oz oat flour

1 tbsp baking powder

A great oat biscuit. Easy to make and ready in a jiffy. My children LOVE these!

1 Preheat the oven to 170°C/325°F/Gas Mark 3.

2 Heat 4 tbsp of olive oil, 4 tbsp of nut oil, 4 tbsp of clear honey and 115g/4 oz pure cane sugar in a pan.

3 Stir in 85g/3 oz oats, 55g/2 oz unsweetened desiccated coconut and 115g/4 oz oat flour.

4 Dissolve 1 tbsp of baking powder in 1 tbsp of hot water and add to the mixture.

5 Take the pan off the heat to cool.

6 Roll the mixture into golf size balls then press each down on to a baking tray. Add 1 to 2 tbsp of honey to the mixture if it is not sticking together well.

7 Place in the oven for 12 minutes.

NOTES

Gingerbread Fingers

Ingredients
Makes 10 to 12 fingers

340g/12 oz rye flour

pinch baking powder

1 tsp ground ginger

zest and juice of ½ lemon

200g/7 oz pure cane sugar

3 tbsp clear honey

4 tbsp grape seed oil

4 tbsp olive oil plus some for lining tray

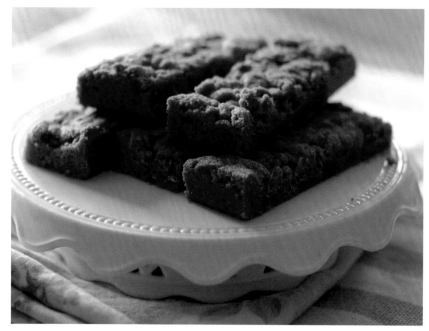

My grandfather-in-law, Eric, loves sweet treats and after acquiring his 'Gingerbread Fingers' recipe, I have made this slightly healthier version.

NOTES

1   Preheat the oven to 150°C/300°F/Gas Mark 2.

2   Mix 340g/12 oz rye flour, a pinch of baking powder, 1 tsp of ground ginger and the zest of ½ a lemon in a bowl.

3   In a saucepan warm 200g/7 oz pure cane sugar, the juice of ½ a lemon, 3 tbsp of clear honey, 4 tbsp of grape seed oil and 4 tbsp of olive oil.

4   Add the liquid to the bowl and stir well until you have a crumble mixture.

5   Stir 2 tbsp of water into the mixture.

6   Line a rectangular baking tin with olive oil and then greaseproof paper and press the mix down with the back of a fork. Score lightly into fingers and bake for approximately 25 to 30 minutes.

7   Once cooked and still warm, score into fingers and leave to cool and harden.

Stewed Fruit

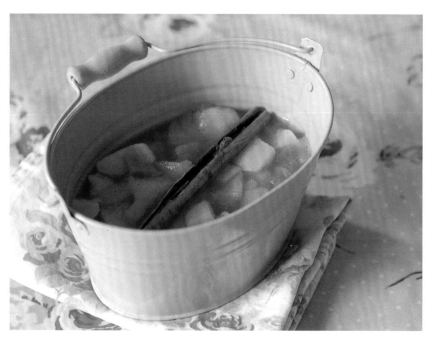

You can add a good selection of fruits in this recipe to make a delicious dessert.

Stewed Fresh Fruit *Serves 4*

Ingredients

800g/28 oz fresh fruit: pineapple, apples, plums, apricots and peaches

150g/5 oz pure cane sugar

2 tsp lemon juice

pinch of mixed spice and ground nutmeg

1 cinnamon stick

Stewed Dried Fruit *Serves 4*

Ingredients

dried apples, apricots, cranberries, currants and any other fruit of your choice

115g/4 oz pure cane sugar

¼ tsp ground cinnamon

¼ tsp ground nutmeg

¼ tsp mixed spice

115g/4 oz chopped walnuts, almonds or pecans

NOTES

1 *Fresh fruit:* Weigh out 800g/28 oz of peeled and quartered fresh fruit, which could include pineapple, apples, plums, apricots and peaches.

2 Mix 150g/5 oz cane sugar (reduce the sugar for a less sweet sauce), 50ml/2 fl oz water and 2 tsp lemon juice in a casserole dish. Add a pinch of mixed spice, ground nutmeg and a cinnamon stick. Carefully stir in fruit.

3 Cover and microwave for 8 to 12 minutes, stirring once during cooking. Or cook on the hob in a large pan. Cover with the lid and bring to boil. Then turn the heat down and simmer for 30 minutes.

4 *Dried fruit:* Place a couple of handfuls of a mix of your choice of: dried apples, apricots, cranberries or currants, etc into a saucepan. Add 115g/4 oz pure cane sugar, a ¼ of a tsp each of cinnamon, nutmeg and mixed spice. Top with 115g/4 oz chopped walnuts, almonds or pecans.

5 Cover the fruit with ½ inch of water. Put a lid on the saucepan and bring to boil, cooking until tender.

6 Serve this on its own, with a dollop of natural yoghurt or with *Buckwheat Pancakes (page 17).*

Baked Apples

Ingredients *Serves 4*

4 large cooking apples

100g/4 oz pure cane sugar

1 tsp ground cinnamon

50ml/2 fl oz grape seed oil

50g/2 oz sultanas

50g/2 oz dried berries-
cranberries, blueberries and
other berries of your choice

25g/1 oz pecan nuts or
flaked almonds

4 tbsp pure apple juice

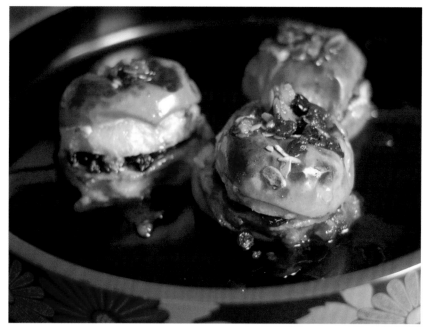

People often like a break from heavy desserts when they come over for dinner. These look good and show a lot of effort in the making!

NOTES

1   Preheat the oven to 190°C/375°F/Gas Mark 5.

2   Core 4 large cooking apples with a small knife, leaving about 0.5cm/0.2 inches uncut at the bottom.

3   Run the tip of the sharp knife round the circumference of each apple and cut in half.

4   Combine 100g/4 oz pure cane sugar, 1 tsp of cinnamon, 50ml/2 fl oz grape seed oil, 50g/2 oz sultanas and 50g/2 oz mixed berries in a bowl. (Try to use cranberries and blueberries and any other berries of your choice).

5   Take the top off the apple and pile the mixture inside.

6   Place the tops on and scatter over 25g/1 oz pecan nuts or flaked almonds. Cook in a dish for 25 to 35 minutes, drizzling over 4 tbsp of pure apple juice and juices from the bottom of the dish, while cooking. This will prevent the apples from drying out.

Pears with Pecan and Cranberries

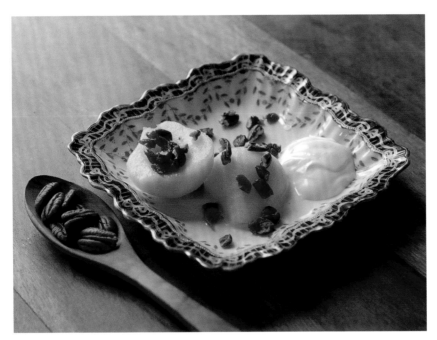

Ingredients *Serves 1*

1 pear

½ tsp pure cane sugar

¼ lemon

handful dried cranberries

handful pecan nuts

dollop natural yoghurt

This is one of my favourite desserts for its simplicity – it is sooooo quick and easy and dinner guests love it!

1   Peel and halve one pear and scoop out the core.

2   Place in a microwaveable dish and cover the pear with ½ tsp of pure cane sugar, the juice of a ¼ of a lemon and a handful of dried cranberries.

3   Cover the dish with cling film and place in the microwave for 3 minutes until the pear is soft.

4   Break up a handful of pecan nuts and sprinkle over the pear.

5   Serve with natural yoghurt.

NOTES

Coconut Milk Smoothie

Ingredients *Serves 4*

300g/11 oz frozen
raspberries or blueberries

2 ripe bananas

350ml/12 fl oz coconut milk

2 tbsp honey

handful fresh mint

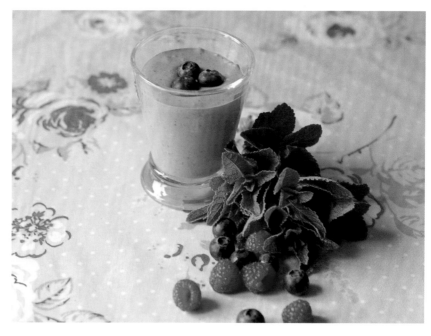

*The addition of coconut milk make this one creamy smoothie/dessert.
Absolutely amazing!*

NOTES

1   Blend 300g/11 oz frozen raspberries or blueberries, 2 ripe bananas, 350ml/12 fl oz coconut milk, 2 tbsp of honey and a handful of mint if desired.

2   Pour the smoothie into the glasses and leave to set for a short time before serving.

Mango Ice

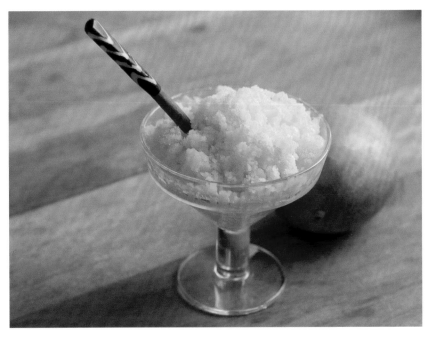

Ingredients *Serves 2 to 4*

1 mango

50ml/2 fl oz pure apple juice

200g/7 oz tinned lychee in natural juices

A great choice for a palette cleanser. Take out of the freezer 20 minutes before serving, so just firm enough to break it up but not too slushy.

1 Peel 1 mango and put the flesh into a blender with 50ml/2 fl oz pure apple juice and 200g/7oz of canned lychees with their natural juices.

2 Pour into a shallow dish and freeze for a couple of hours.

3 Take out of the freezer 20 minutes before serving and use a fork to break up the ice. Serve in cocktail glasses.

NOTES

SAUCES AND BREADS MOVING FORWARD

*Healthy sauces are an invaluable addition to a meal. When it comes to bread, spelt, corn, pumpernickel, buckwheat and rye bread are all good healthy alternatives to white bread. Your healthfood shop should stock them. Try making your own bread. The Rye Bread recipe can be used from Day 26 in **the 28 Day Plan**.*

Tomato and Vegetable Sauce

Ingredients *Serves 6*

2 tbsp olive oil

1 courgette

1 red pepper

1 carrot

1 small onion

800g/28 oz tinned tomatoes

2 garlic cloves

2 tbsp natural vegetable stock powder

NOTES

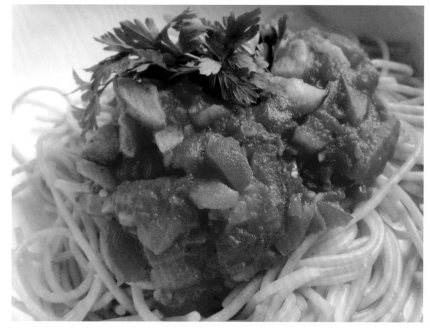

This is a simple and nutritious sauce for children. You can blend the sauce if they don't like lumps! Good with pasta or meat.

1 Heat 2 tbsp of olive oil in a large saucepan.

2 Finely chop 1 courgette, 1 red pepper, 1 carrot and 1 small onion and add to the frying pan. Cook until softened.

3 Add 800g/28 oz tinned tomatoes, 2 crushed garlic cloves and 2 tbsp of natural vegetable stock powder. Stir and heat to simmering point.

4 Season with salt and pepper.

5 Simmer for 10 minutes and serve.

Rye Bread

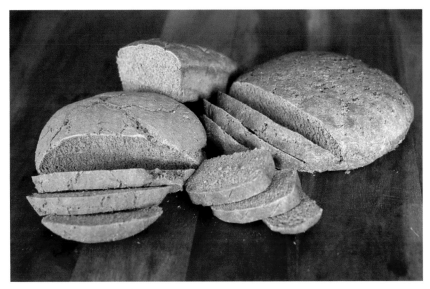

Ingredients *Makes 2 loaves*

400g/14 oz rye flour

500g/17.5 oz spelt flour

1.5 tsp yeast

600ml/20 fl oz warm water

*(3 tbsp honey)

use honey after the 28 day plan

This is great bread with a bit of smoked fish on top. Use this recipe from Day 26 of the 28 Day Plan.

1 Put 400g/14 oz rye flour, 500g/17.5 oz spelt flour, 1.5 tsp yeast and 1 tsp salt into a large sized mixing bowl and mix well. Add 3 tbsp honey (after the 28 day plan) to 600ml/20 fl oz warm water and stir to dissolve. Then pour into the flour and yeast.

2 Mix to form a sticky dough, tip onto a floured board or work surface. Stretch and knead the dough for about 5 minutes, then form into a ball. Lightly oil the bowl and put the dough ball back in. Cover with a tea towel and place in a warm place for about an hour.

3 At this stage you have two options. Either remove the dough from the bowl and knead it again for a minute. Divide the dough in half and place in the prepared loaf tins. Cover again with a tea towel and set aside for a further 30 minutes until risen. Set the oven at 220°C/425 °F/Gas Mark 7. Bake for 30 minutes, until slightly crispy on top. Remove from the oven and leave in its tin for 10 minutes. Take it out of its tin to cool down further.

4 Or you can leave the dough for 2 hours and place it on a oiled baking sheet as it is, in the oven for the same time as mentioned in point 3.

5 You may notice that the loaf with honey comes out a little darker in colour than the loaf without.

NOTES

Olive Bread

Ingredients *Makes 1 loaf*

650g/23 oz spelt flour

2 tsp yeast

2 tbsp pure cane sugar

125g/4 oz pitted black olives

3 tbsp olive oil

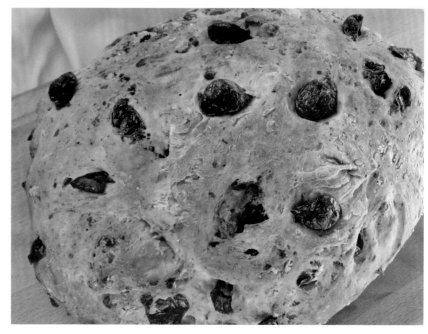

This never lasts very long in our house!

NOTES

1 Mix together in a large bowl 650g/23 oz spelt flour, 2 tsp of yeast, 2 tbsp of pure cane sugar, 1 tsp of salt, 125g/4 oz pitted black olives, 3 tbsp of olive oil and 300ml/11 fl oz warm water.

2 Knead on a floured board for 5 minutes and cover and leave to rise for 2 hours.

3 Preheat the oven to 240°C/475°F/Gas Mark 9.

4 Gently turn the loaf out on to a baking sheet that has been lightly oiled. Bake the loaf in the oven for 15 minutes.

5 Lower the baking tray and reduce heat to 190°C/375°F/Gas Mark 5 for another 15 minutes, or until done.

Mixed Seed Bread

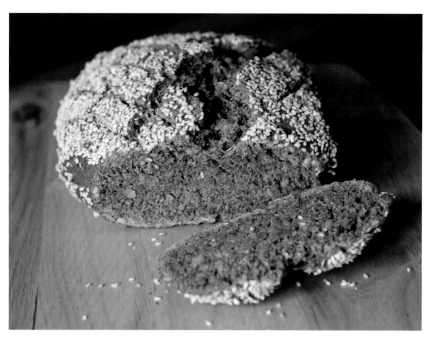

Ingredients *Makes 1 loaf*

400g/14 oz spelt flour

100g/4 oz rye flour

2 tsp yeast

125g/4 oz sunflower seeds

50g/2 oz poppy seeds

75g/3 oz molasses

50g/2 oz sesame seeds

Not only does this Mixed Seed Bread taste good but is really fun to make!

1 Mix 400g/14 oz spelt flour, 100g/4 oz rye flour, 2 tsp of salt, 2 tsp of yeast, 125g/4 oz sunflower seeds and 50g/2 oz poppy seeds in a large bowl.

2 Add 75g/3 oz molasses and 300ml/11 fl oz water. If the dough is still dry, add another tablespoon of water.

3 Knead on a floured board for 5 minutes.

4 Put back in a lightly oiled bowl, cover and leave somewhere warm for 2 hours.

5 Preheat the oven to 220°C/425°F/Gas Mark 7.

6 Roll the dough in 50g/2 oz sesame seeds and then cut the top into criss-cross slashes with a sharp knife.

7 Bake for 30 minutes until the loaf sounds hollow when tapped underneath. Cool on a wire rack.

NOTES

Cinnamon Raisin Bread

Ingredients *Makes 1 loaf*

130g/5 oz spelt flour

130g/5 oz rye flour

50g/2 oz pure cane sugar

1 tbsp baking powder

1 tbsp cinnamon

2 eggs

200ml/7 fl oz rice milk

95ml/3 fl oz grape seed oil plus for lining tin

130g/5 oz raisins

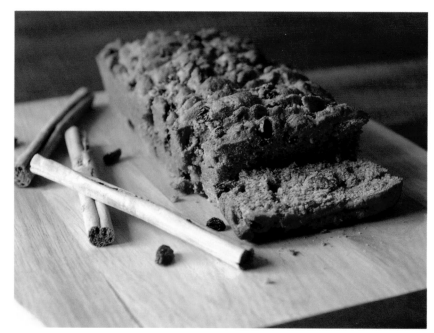

This is good to serve in the afternoon with a cuppa.

1   Preheat the oven to 180°C/350°F/Gas Mark 4.

2   Grease a loaf tin with grape seed oil and and a sprinkle of spelt flour.

3   In a large bowl, stir in 130g/5 oz spelt flour, 130g/5 oz rye flour, 50g/2 oz pure cane sugar, a ¼ of a tsp of salt, 1 tbsp of baking powder and 1 tbsp of cinnamon.

4   In a small bowl, beat 2 eggs.

5   Add 200ml/7 fl oz rice milk and 95 ml/3 fl oz grape seed oil to the small bowl and mix.

6   Add the contents of the small bowl to the large bowl.

7   Combine until just blended and add 130g/5 oz raisins. Place the mixture into the loaf tin and bake for 45 minutes or until done.

8   Cool in the tin for 10 minutes and then turn out on to a wire rack. Lovely toasted and served with a cup of tea!

TIPS ON HAVING A DINNER PARTY

Menu example

HORS D'OEUVRES

If you are following the 28 Day Plan prepare something you can eat too, such as carrot and cucumber sticks with a either of the following:

Guacamole Dip (V): Mash together 2 avocados, 1 crushed garlic clove, 1 large tomato (skinned), the juice of 1 lemon, a dash of salt (and a splash of tabasco after the 28 day plan!).

Make your own *Houmous (V):* Soak 400g/14 oz chickpeas overnight and boil for 30 minutes and drain (or use a can of chickpeas).

Add a generous glug of olive oil to the chickpeas, juice of ½ lemon, 1 tsp salt, ¼ tsp pepper and 1 or 2 crushed garlic cloves and mix together using an electric mixer. Add more oil if the paste is very stiff. Blend in a handful of mint leaves for *Minted Houmous*.

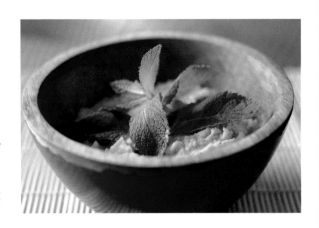

STARTER

Smoked Salmon and Grapefruit (p49) *or* PeaSoup (p21)

PALETTE CLEANSER

Mango Ice (p95) after the 28 day plan

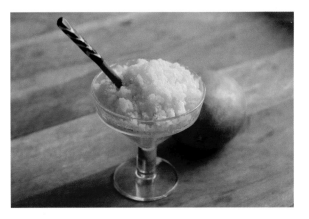

MAIN COURSE

Stuffed Squash (p32) *or* Spicy Lamb with Warm Quinoa (p71) after the 28 day plan

DESSERT

Baked Pineapples (p54) *or* Blueberry and Cinnamon Cake (p83) after the 28 day plan

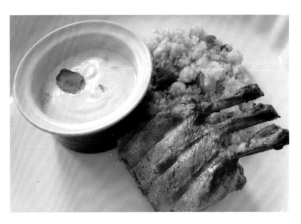

SHOPPING LISTS

Cut out or photocopy the shopping list to make food shopping easier

Breakfast *28 day plan*

	Serves				
'Smooth' smoothie (p14)		½ grapefruit	1 lime	5 apples/or 120ml/4 fl oz apple juice	
'Tangy' smoothie (p14)		1 lemon	1 lime	½ small pineapple	5 apples/or 120ml/4 fl oz apple juice
'Refreshing' smoothie (p14)		1 apple	2 oranges	10 mint leaves	
'Filling' smoothie (p14)		¼ cucumber	10 mint leaves	9 apples/or 220ml/7 fl oz apple juice	
'Sweet' smoothie (p14)		½ small pineapple	1 lime	5 apples/or 120ml/4 fl oz apple juice	(½ a grapefruit)
'Creamy' smoothie (p14)		½ melon	9 apples/or 220ml/7 fl oz apple juice		
'1' Juice (p14)		4 oranges	1 apple	large handful lamb's lettuce	
'2' Juice (p14)		3 apples	½ yellow pepper	4 large lettuce leaves	handful of mint
'3' Juice (p14)		4 oranges	2 large carrots	1 tsp fresh ginger	handful of mint
Fruit Parfait (p15)	Serves 1	a handful of fresh fruit	2 tbsp natural yoghurt	sprinkle of either barley or oat bran	
Grapefruit (p15)	Serves 1	sprinkle of ground almonds	½ grapefruit	sprinkle of hemp seed	(boiled egg)
Melon (p15)	Serves 1	½ a melon	sprinkle of seeds	sprinkle of almonds	
Fruit Salad (p15)		fruits of your choice	hemp seeds	berries	

Millet Porridge (p17)	Serves 2	75g/3 oz millet flakes	(or 75g/3 oz buckwheat flakes)	(or 75g/3 oz barley flakes)	(or 75g/3 oz oat flakes)	ground cinnamon	grated apple	seeds including hemp	berries
		nuts	live yoghurt	rice, oat, spelt or almond milk to taste					
Buckwheat Pancakes (p17)	Makes 6	100g/3 oz buckwheat flour	1 egg	Choice of fillings:	salmon, eggs	salmon, natural live yoghurt, paprika	chicken, salad	watercress, avocado	coconut oil
Mackerel (p15)	Serves 1	1 mackerel (fillet)	fruit						
Scrambled Egg (p15)	Serves 1	1 or 2 eggs	5 cherry tomatoes						
Omelette (p15)	Serves 1	1 egg	1 small onion	1 mushroom	mint leaves	salmon streaks	handful spinach leaves	olive oil	(goat's cheese)
En Cocotte (p17)	Serves 1	olive oil	1 tsp freshly chopped thyme	2 tbsp natural yoghurt	2 eggs				
Fried Breakfast (p15)	Serves 1	olive oil	2 eggs	a handful of mushrooms	4 cherry tomatoes				

Lunch or Dinner 28 day plan

Butternut Squash Soup (p18)	Serves 4	1.5kg/3.3 lbs butternut squash	2 tbsp olive oil	1 onion	2 garlic cloves	1 tsp nutmeg	¼ tsp curry powder	240ml/8 fl oz freshly squeezed apple juice (approx 2 large apples)	
Carrot Soup (p19)	Serves 4	2 onions	2 garlic cloves	6 carrots	2 celery stalks	1 tbsp natural veg stock powder	herbs of your choice	100g/4 oz ground almonds	
Lentil Soup (p20)	Serves 4	200g/7 oz puy lentils	2 tbsp natural veg stock powder	1 onion	100g/4 oz spinach leaves	(marmite)			
Pea Soup (p21)	Serves 4	olive oil	2 large onions	1 celery stick	1 carrot	1 garlic clove	400g/14 oz frozen peas	1 tbsp natural veg stock powder	25g/1 oz fresh basil leaves
Mixed Vegetable and Coconut Milk Soup (p22)	Serves 4	handful fresh coriander	1 onion	4 carrots	1 beetroot	olive oil	240g/8 oz frozen peas	½ cauliflower	2 bay leaves
			1 tbsp natural veg stock powder	240ml/8 fl oz coconut milk					

Aubergine Rolls (p23)	Makes 10	1 aubergine · olive oil · 10 basil leaves · 100g/1.75 oz tempeh · 10 cherry tomatoes
Melon with Parma Ham (p24)	Serves 4	8 slices parma ham · 1 melon (galia, cantaloupe, watermelon or a selection of all three) · 80g rocket · 1 pomegranate · olive oil
Eggy Bread (p25)	Serves 1	olive oil · 1 egg · 50 ml/2 fl oz rice milk · 1 or 2 slices of rye or pumpernickel bread · slices of fresh fruit · (honey)
Grilled Tomatoes (p26)	Serves 1	olive oil · 1 large tomato · 1 slice rye or pumpernickel bread · balsamic vinegar
Soy Mung Bean Sprouts (p27)	Serves 2	2 tbsp olive oil · 1 tbsp soy sauce · 200g/7 oz raw mung bean sprouts · 1 tsp sesame oil · 1 large onion
Thai Curry with Tempeh and Vegetables (p28)	Serves 1	1 small onion · olive oil · 1 garlic clove · 2 tsp curry powder · handful fresh basil · 2 handfuls fresh coriander · 415ml/15 fl oz coconut milk · ½ red pepper · 100g/3.5 oz tempeh · 2 lime wedges
Nutty Mixed Salad (p29)	Serves 1	2 large lettuce leaves · handful of rocket · ¼ pepper · 1 radish · 4 cherry tomatoes · ½ thumb size spring onion · handful cashews, pine nuts, sunflower and poppy seeds · 2 brazil nuts
Salad Dressing (p29)	Serves 1	1 tbsp soy sauce · 1 small garlic clove · olive oil · sprinkle parsley · (1 tsp mustard)
Millet Cauliflower (p30)	Serves 2	150g/5 oz millet · 1 tbsp natural veg stock powder · 1 small cauliflower head · 2 garlic cloves · 1 tsp each of ground cumin, paprika, curry powder · handful fresh parsley · 1 large red onion · 1 dollop natural yoghurt · 60g/2 oz frozen peas
Stuffed Tomatoes (p31)	Serves 2	2 large, relatively hard beef tomatoes · 1 tbsp curry powder · 1 tbsp cumin seed · 250g/9 oz beef mince · 1 tbsp natural beef stock powder · ½ courgette · ½ yellow pepper · ½ onion · ¼ cucumber · 1 tbsp coriander · 1 tbsp lemon juice · 1 tbsp olive oil

Stuffed Squash (p32)	Serves 2	1 butternut squash or pumpkin	½ courgette	½ yellow pepper	½ onion	1 tbsp lemon juice	1 tbsp olive oil	1 tbsp curry powder	flaked soya
		1 tbsp cumin seeds							
Roast Chicken (p33)	Serves 4	1 large chicken	1 lemon	5 garlic cloves	olive oil	a few parsnips, onions, carrots and leeks			
				1 large tomato	handful mint leaves				
Chicken Tikka (p34)	Serves 1	1 chicken breast	300g/11 oz natural yoghurt	1 garlic clove	sprinkle tandoori/tikka or curry powder				
Soy Spinach (p34)	Serves 1	50g/2 oz pine nuts	1 garlic clove	olive oil	2 handfuls fresh spinach	1 tbsp soy sauce			
Green Indian Curry (p35)	Serves 1	1 small onion	1 garlic clove	1 tsp each ground turmeric, ground coriander, ground paprika, ground cumin	1 chicken breast or beef/lamb as an alternative	¼ cauliflower head	small handful green beans	2 carrots	2 tbsp ground almonds
		small handful fresh spinach	fresh coriander	dollop natural yoghurt	handful flaked almonds	olive oil			
Soy Steak (p36)	Serves 1	1 sirloin steak	olive oil	2 garlic cloves	3 tbsp soy sauce	4 mushrooms	1 onion	serve with broccoli or Nutty Mixed Salad (p29)	
Moroccan Beef Stew with Pumpkin (p37)	Serves 2	olive oil	1 large onion	1 garlic clove	2 tsp ground cumin	250g/9 oz stewing beef	2 ripe tomatoes	200g/7 oz pumpkin or butternut squash	1 tbsp natural beef stock powder
		1 bay leaf	3 large plums	2 tbsp ground almonds	fresh coriander	dollop of natural yoghurt			
Meat Balls (p38)	Makes 6 balls	250g/9 oz beef mince	1 red onion	3 garlic cloves	2 tsp dried mixed herbs	3 good sized tomatoes	pinch paprika	12 basil leaves	serve with steamed vegetables or Courgette and Almonds (p39)
Courgette and Almonds (p39)	Serves 2	2 handfuls flaked almonds	olive oil	1 courgette	1 or 2 garlic cloves	(1 onion)			

Burgers (p40)	Makes 4	250g/9 oz beef mince	1 onion	glug of olive oil	sprinkle of dried Italian herbs	fresh coriander	1 egg	1 tbsp tomato purée	serve with Lentil Salad (p41) or Ginger Garlic Green Beans (p42)
Lentil Salad (p41)	Serves 1	50g/2 oz puy lentils	½ red onion	1 tbsp olive oil	1 large tomato	1 lime	4/5 basil leaves	1 egg	
Ginger Garlic Green Beans (p42)	Serves 4	500g/18 oz of green beans	2 tbsp olive oil	1 tsp sesame oil	2 garlic cloves	2.5cm/1 inch fresh ginger	1 tbsp natural chicken stock powder	2 tbsp soy sauce	
Red Bean Burger (p43)	Makes 4	1 tbsp olive oil	1 small onion	1 garlic clove	1 tsp each of ground cumin, ground coriander, ground turmeric	115g/4 oz mushrooms	400g/14 oz kidney beans (or a can)	serve with salad or Ratatouille (p44)	
Ratatouille (p44)	Serves 4	1 aubergine	1 courgette	2 onions	1 yellow or red pepper	3 garlic cloves	7 large tomatoes	handful fresh basil	1 tbsp olive oil
King Prawn Salad (p45)	Serves 1	2 large lettuce leaves	handful rocket	½ avocado	¼ red pepper	6 fresh/frozen king prawns	2 garlic cloves	2 tbsp lemon juice	olive oil
		fresh/dried dill							
Tasty Prawns (p46)	Serves 1	1 garlic clove	1 tsp grated ginger	handful fresh coriander	½ tsp cumin seeds	a sprinkle of curry powder	handful fresh parsley	1 tbsp lemon juice	150g/5 oz pot natural yoghurt
		8 fresh, uncooked king prawns or 1 chicken breast	olive or coconut oil	120g/4 oz of mung bean sprouts					
Salmon with Cucumber and Pomegranate Salad (p47)	Serves 1	1 salmon steak	olive oil	1 garlic clove	½ tsp paprika	½ cucumber	½ pomegranate	1 spring onion	handful cherry tomatoes
		large handful fresh mint	2 limes						
Roasted Salmon with Pesto (p48)	Serves 1	1 salmon fillet	½ lemon	½ red pepper	¼ courgette	1-2 tbsp flaked soya	Pesto sauce (p59)	mixed herbs	serve with peas or roasted tomatoes or Coriander and Cherry tomatoes (p48)

Coriander and Cherry Tomatoes (p48)	Serves 1	2 tbsp olive oil	8 cherry tomatoes	handful fresh coriander	(2 tsp mirin)				parsley or coriander
Smoked Salmon and Grapefruit (p49)	Serves 1	½ grapefruit	1 avocado	1 tbsp olive oil	1 tsp balsamic vinegar	½ lemon	4 smoked salmon slices	handful of lettuce leaves	serve with ½ small broccoli or Roasted Vegetables (p52)
Baked Fish Fillet (p50)	Serves 1	1 piece of meaty white fish	2 garlic cloves	1 tbsp olive oil	1 tsp lemon juice	small handful fresh parsley and chives	pinch paprika	2 slices from a large tomato	
Fried Fish (p51)	Serves 1	1 or 2 pieces of white fish	1 tbsp olive oil	2 lettuce leaves	2 cherry tomatoes	4 olives	a handful of chopped yellow and red peppers	(spelt flour)	
Roasted Vegetables (p52)	Serves 1	½ courgette	½ red pepper	1 onion	2 tbsp fresh herbs of your choice	1 tbsp olive oil	1 garlic clove		
Fish Cakes (p53)	Serves 2	150g/5 oz salmon meat	150g/5 oz crab meat	handful fresh coriander	½ spring onion	olive oil			
Cucumber Salsa (p53)	Serves 2	¼ cucumber	handful fresh coriander	½ lime	dollop natural yoghurt	(½ red chili)			

Desserts 28 day plan

Lollies (p54)		fresh juice	lolly moulds			
Baked Pineapples (p54)	Serves 1	2 pineapple rings or 1 pineapple	sprinkle of chilli powder	2 tbsp ground cinnamon	absorbent paper	(20g/1 oz pure cane sugar)
Stewed Orange (p54)	Serves 1	1 orange				

Sauces and Toppings 28 day plan

Lemon Dressing (p58)	Serves 4	150g/5 oz natural yoghurt	1 tbsp olive oil	1 tbsp nut oil	2 tbsp lemon juice	¼ tsp grated lemon rind	2 tbsp fresh chives
Peanut Butter Sauce (p56)	Serves 4	5 tbsp smooth peanut butter	2 tbsp soy sauce	1 tsp ground coriander	1 tsp ground cumin	1 lime	150ml/5 fl oz coconut milk

Herb Topping for Fish (p57)	Serves 4	2 tbsp of nuts of your choice (walnut, cashew, brazil, almond); 8 tbsp flaked soya	2 tbsp fresh dill	2 tbsp fresh parsley	2 tbsp fresh chives	6 plum tomatoes	200g/7 oz natural yoghurt	1 lemon	2 tbsp olive oil
Curry Yoghurt Sauce (p58)	Serves 4	1 tsp curry powder	150g/5 oz pot of natural yoghurt	a handful of fresh mint	2 tbsp olive oil				
Pesto (p59)	Serves 6-8	125g/4 oz fresh basil leaves	2 garlic cloves	100g/4 oz pine nuts	200ml/7 fl oz olive oil				
Simple Spinach Sauce (p60)	Serves 4	200g/7 oz fresh spinach	1 tbsp natural veg stock powder	2 garlic cloves	olive oil				

Snacks 28 day plan

Vegetable Sticks and Houmous (p61)	Serves 4	400g/14 oz chickpeas (or a can)	1 or 2 garlic cloves	juice ½ lemon	2 carrots	½ cucumber	olive oil	(mint leaves)
Vegetable Sticks and Guacamole (p61)	Serves 4	2 avocados	1 garlic clove	1 large tomato	1 lemon	(splash tabasco)	2 carrots	½ cucumber
Carrot Sticks and Peanut Butter (p61)	Serves 1	1 carrot stick	2 tbsp pure peanut butter					
Melon/ Grapefruit with Nuts and Seeds (p61)	Serves 1	¼ melon/ ½ grapefruit	handful hemp seeds or almonds					
Fruit with Chicken (p61)	Serves 1	Fruit of your choice	2 slices chicken					
Seaweed and Tempeh (p61)	Serves 1	½ sheet dried nori	2 cubes tempeh	splash soy sauce				
Fruit and Nuts (p61)	Serves 1	Fruit and nuts of your choice						
Salmon and Yoghurt (p61)	Serves 1	Slice of salmon	1 tbsp natural yoghurt	1 lettuce leaf	sprinkle paprika			

Stewed Orange and Prawns (p61)	Serves 1	1 orange	handful cooked prawns						
Melon and Parma Ham (p61)	Serves 1	2 slices melon	2 slices parma ham						

Breakfast Moving Forward

Peanut Banana Smoothie (p62)	Serves 1	1 banana	3 tbsp of natural yoghurt	125ml/4 fl oz rice milk	1 tbsp peanut butter	1 tsp runny honey			
Summer Fruits Smoothie (p63)	Serves 4	1 old banana (frozen)	200g/7 oz frozen mixed fruits	200g/7 oz natural yoghurt	500ml/18 fl oz rice milk	honey			
Mini Frittatas (p64)	Makes 15	olive oil	1/3 courgette	1/3 red pepper	4 eggs	150ml/5 fl oz rice milk	1 tbsp freshly chopped thyme	150g/5 oz goat's cheese	muffin tray
Pineapple and Carrot Muffins (p65)	Makes 12	200g/7 oz spelt flour	2 tsp baking powder	2 tsp cinnamon	50ml/2 fl oz grape seed oil	50ml/2 fl oz rice milk	90g/3 oz pure cane sugar	2 eggs	120g/4 oz carrots
		225g/8 oz crushed pineapple							
Honey Drenched Nuts (p66)		nuts of your choice (unsalted cashew, walnut, whole almonds, brazil, pecan, macadamia, sunflower)	glass jar	clear honey					
Oat Surprise (p67)	Serves 1	1/4 apple	2 tbsp apple compote	20g/1 oz oats	handful frozen berries				

Lunch or Dinner Moving Forward

Coconut Millet Salad (p68)	Serves 4	250g/9 oz millet	1 tbsp of natural vegetable stock powder	175g/6 oz ready to eat soft dried apricots	small bunch fresh chives	2 tbsp unsweetened desiccated coconut	1/2 tsp cinnamon	1 tbsp olive oil	juice of 1/2 an orange
		1/2 tsp finely grated orange rind	1 tsp wholegrain mustard	1 tsp clear honey	2 tbsp fresh mint				

Vegetable Stir Fry (p69)	Serves 4	3 tbsp nut oil	3 tbsp of sesame oil	3 garlic cloves	2.5cm/1 inch fresh ginger	3 carrots	350g/12 oz broccoli florets	250g/9 oz asparagus tips	2 large spring onions
		300g/11 oz Chinese leaf	4 tbsp soy sauce	3 tbsp mirin	1 tbsp sesame seeds	4 baby corn	peanut butter sauce (p56) if desired		
Chicken and Rice (p70)	Serves 4	500g/17.5 oz wild or brown rice	olive oil	4 chicken thighs	2 onions	2 garlic cloves	1 tbsp tomato purée	1 tsp paprika	1 tbsp natural chicken stock powder
		1 tbsp wholegrain mustard	dollop natural yoghurt	1 yellow pepper	1 red pepper				
Spicy Lamb with Warm Quinoa (p71)	Serves 4	250g/9 oz quinoa	handful rocket	1 lemon	1 tbsp natural chicken stock powder	1 tsp mild chilli powder	3 tsp curry powder	olive oil	500g/17 oz natural yoghurt
		a rack of lamb weighing approx 600g/21 oz	handful fresh mint	400g/14 oz chickpeas or a can					
Beef Curry with Pumpkin and Prunes (p72)	Serves 4 to 6	2 large onions	2 garlic cloves	2 tsp ground cumin	2 tsp curry powder	800g/28 oz stewing beef	4 ripe tomatoes	600g/21 oz pumpkin	2 tbsp natural beef stock powder
		2 bay leaves	3 handfuls pitted prunes	3 tbsp ground almonds	500g/18 oz pot of natural yoghurt	brown rice	olive oil	handful of fresh coriander	
BBQ Orange Duck (p73)	Serves 4	370g/13 oz marmalade (100% fruit spread)	4 duck breasts	4 tbsp runny honey	serve with Courgette and Almonds (p39) and/or Coconut Millet Salad (p68)				
Spaghetti Bolognese (p74)	Serves 4	2 tsp olive oil	2 garlic cloves	1 onion	1 carrot	500g/18 oz beef mince	200g/7 oz mushrooms	2 tsp Italian herbs	1 tsp oregano
		3 good-sized tomatoes (or a 400g can)	2 tbsp tomato purée	2 tsp Worcestershire sauce	handful fresh basil leaves	50ml/2 fl oz rice milk	wholewheat or spelt pasta		
Vegetarian Bolognese (p74)	Serves 4	2 tsp olive oil	2 garlic cloves	1 onion	1 carrot	2 x 200g/7 oz pack tempeh	200g/7 oz mushrooms	2 tsp Italian herbs	1 tsp oregano
		3 tomatoes (or a 400g can)	2 tbsp tomato purée	2 tsp Worcestershire sauce	handful fresh basil leaves	50ml/2 fl oz rice milk	wholewheat or spelt pasta		

Meaty Fish with Japanese Sauce (p75)	Serves 2	2 pieces of swordfish	1 lemon	olive oil	1 tbsp pure cane sugar	1 tbsp mirin or fish sauce	1 tbsp soy sauce	serve with handful of beans or broccoli or Raw Broccoli Salad (p76)	
Raw Broccoli Salad (p76)	Serves 4	100g/4 oz flaked almonds	500g/18 oz natural yoghurt	500g/18 oz broccoli florets	160g/6 oz raisins	40g/1 oz sultanas			
Sardine Pasta (p77)	Serves 4	200g/7 oz wholewheat or spelt pasta	½ fennel	2 tbsp olive oil	100g/4 oz frozen peas	125g/4 oz frozen sweetcorn	125g/4 oz tin sardines	4 chopped anchovies	handful capers
		2 handfuls pine nuts	handful fresh parsley						
Oriental Grilled Tuna Steaks (p78)	Serves 2	2 tuna steaks	1 spring onion	25ml/1 fl oz mirin	25ml/1 fl oz soy sauce	6 tbsp coconut oil or olive oil	1 tbsp grated ginger	serve with brown rice, green beans or Soy Mung Bean Sprouts (p27)	handful dry or fresh seaweed
Creamy Pumpkin Soup (p79)	Serves 4	1kg/2.2lbs pumpkin	1 onion	2 tbsp olive oil	½ tsp nutmeg	½ tsp pure cane sugar	2 tbsp natural veg stock powder		
Quick Salad Dressing (p80)		olive oil	mirin or (or clear honey)	soy sauce	mixed herbs to taste (dried or fresh)	1 tbsp pure cane sugar			
Caramelized Onions (p81)	Serves 4	1 tbsp olive oil	2 medium red onions	2 medium white onions					
Honey-Glazed Carrots (p82)	Serves 4	450g/16 oz carrots	1 garlic clove	2 tbsp fresh rosemary leaves	1 tbsp nut oil	2 tbsp olive oil	2 tbsp clear honey	1 tbsp lemon juice	

Desserts *Moving Forward*

Blueberry and Cinnamon Cake (p83)	Serves 6	olive oil for lining the tray plus 4 tbsp	4 tbsp nut oil	140g/5 oz pure cane sugar	140g/5 oz ground almonds	140g/5 oz buckwheat flour	3 eggs	1 tsp ground cinnamon plus for dusting	2 tsp vanilla extract
		225g/8 oz blueberries							
Grape Cake (p84)	Serves 6 to 8	450g/16 oz seedless black grapes	225g/8 oz spelt flour plus for dusting grapes	140g/5 oz pure cane sugar	1 tsp baking powder	5 eggs	2 tbsp grape seed oil plus for lining the tray		
Lemon Drizzle (p85)	Serves 6 to 8	4 tbsp grape seed oil	310g/11 oz pure cane sugar	4 eggs	140g/5 oz spelt flour	2 lemons			

Honey Cake (p86)	Serves 6 to 8	175g/6 oz clear honey plus 1 tbsp	3 tbsp olive oil	2 tsp baking powder	95g/3 oz pure cane sugar	2 eggs		200g/7 oz oat flour (or put oats in a blender to make oat flour)	50ml/2 fl oz grape seed oil plus for lining the tray
Avocado Bread Cake (p87)	Serves 8	50ml/2 fl oz grape seed oil	200g/7 oz pure cane sugar plus 25g/1 oz sugar for topping	2 eggs	2 bananas	1 avocado	2 handfuls pecan nuts (plus 5 for decoration)	300g/10 oz spelt flour	2 tsp baking powder
			greaseproof paper		rice milk in reserve				
Oat Spice Cake (p88)	Serves 9 to 12	85g/3 oz oats	1 tbsp nut oil	200g/7 oz pure cane sugar plus 4 tbsp for topping	3 eggs	100g/4 oz spelt flour	½ tsp baking powder	2 tbsp ground cinnamon, plus 2 tsp for topping	1 tsp nutmeg
		grape seed oil for lining tray	½ tsp vanilla extract	40g/1 oz pecan nuts	sprinkle of unsweetened desiccated coconut				
Oat Biscuits (p89)	Makes approx 10-12	4 tbsp olive oil	4 tbsp clear honey (plus 1 to 2 in reserve)	115g/4 oz pure cane sugar	85g/3 oz oats	55g/2 oz unsweetened desiccated coconut		115g/4 oz oat flour (or put oats in a blender to make oat flour)	1 tbsp baking powder
Gingerbread Fingers (p90)	Makes 10 to 12	340g/12 oz rye flour	pinch baking powder	1 tsp ground ginger	½ lemon	200g/7 oz pure cane sugar	3 tbsp clear honey	4 tbsp grape seed oil	4 tbsp olive oil plus for lining the tray
Stewed Fresh Fruit (p91)	Serves 4	800g/28 oz fresh fruit: pineapple, apples, plums, apricots, peaches	150g/5 oz pure cane sugar	2 tsp lemon juice	pinch of mixed spice	pinch of nutmeg	1 cinnamon stick		
Stewed Dried Fruit (p91)	Serves 4	2 handfuls including: dried apples, apricots, cranberries, currants and any other fruit of your choice	115g/4 oz pure cane sugar	¼ tsp ground cinnamon	¼ tsp nutmeg	¼ tsp mixed spice	115g/4 oz chopped walnuts, almonds or pecans		
Baked Apples (p92)	Serves 4	4 large cooking apples	100g/4 oz pure cane sugar	1 tsp ground cinnamon	50ml/2 fl oz grape seed oil	50g/2 oz sultanas	50g/2 oz dried berries—cranberries, blueberries and other berries of your choice	25g/1 oz pecan nuts or flaked almonds	4 tbsp pure apple juice

Pears with Pecan and Cranberries (p93)	Serves 1	1 pear	½ tsp pure cane sugar	¼ of a lemon	handful dried cranberries	handful pecan nuts	dollop natural yoghurt		
Coconut Milk Smoothie (p94)	Serves 4	300g/11 oz frozen raspberries or blueberries	2 ripe bananas	350ml/12 fl oz coconut milk	2 tbsp honey	handful fresh mint if desired			
Mango Ice (p95)	Serves 2-4	1 mango	50ml/2 fl oz pure apple juice	200g/7 oz tinned lychee in natural juices					

Sauces and Breads *Moving Forward*

Tomato and Vegetable Sauce (p96)	Serves 6	2 tbsp olive oil	1 courgette	1 red pepper	1 carrot	1 small onion	800g/28 oz tinned tomatoes	2 garlic cloves	2 tbsp of natural vegetable stock powder
Rye Bread (p97) *(use from Day 26)*	Makes 2 loaves	400g/14 oz rye flour	500g/17.5 oz spelt flour	1.5 tsp yeast	*(3 tbsp honey)				
Olive Bread (p98)	Makes 1 loaf	650g/23 oz spelt flour	2 tsp yeast	2 tbsp pure cane sugar	125g/4 oz pitted black olives	3 tbsp olive oil			
Mixed Seed Bread (p99)	Makes 1 loaf	400g/14 oz spelt flour	2 tsp yeast	125g/4 oz sunflower seeds		50g/2 oz poppy seeds	75g/3 oz molasses	50g/2 oz sesame seeds	
Cinnamon Raisin Bread (p100)	Makes 1 loaf	130g/5 oz spelt flour	130g/5 oz rye flour	50g/2 oz pure cane sugar	1 tbsp baking powder	1 tbsp cinnamon	2 eggs	200ml/7 fl oz rice milk	95ml/3 fl oz grape seed oil + for lining the tin
		130g/5 oz raisins							

Dinner Party *Moving Forward*

Guacamole Dip (V) (p101)	Serves 4	2 avocados	1 garlic clove	1 large tomato	1 lemon	(splash Tabasco)			
Houmous (V) (p101)	Serves 4	400g/14 oz chickpeas (or a can)	olive oil	1 or 2 garlic cloves	(mint leaves)	the juice of half a lemon			

Recipe Index

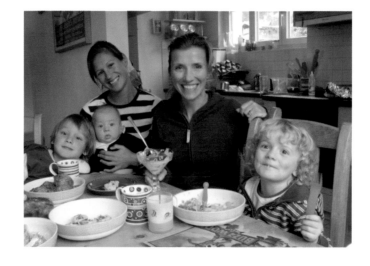

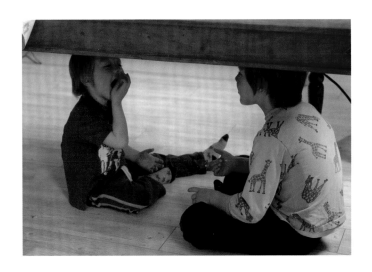

Also by Joey Bull

Joey writes a monthly column for Ultra-FIT Magazine and contributes regularly to Muscle & Fitness Magazine.

She has released five workout DVDs through IMC Vision Ltd:

Ballet Pilates: Ballates Workout

The Body Reshape Plan

Ballet Workout: Total Body Toning

Ballet Workout for Legs, Bums & Tums

10 Minute Method Workouts for Back Pain & Posture

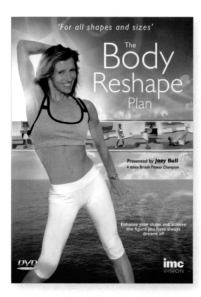
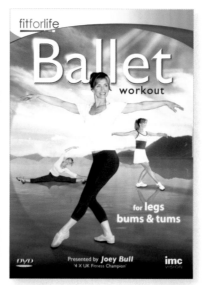
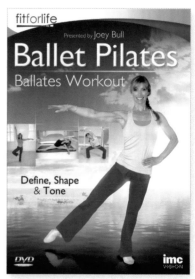

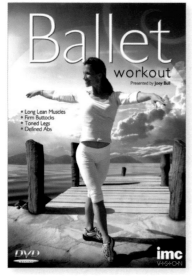
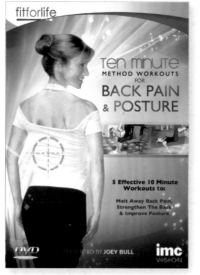

Available through all usual online outlets and from www.imcvision.com.

POSTSCRIPT

In the final stages of completing this book, I was blessed with my baby girl Ottilie. Edward cannot be directly replaced of course, but at my age and after the traumas my body suffered during and after the loss of Edward, she really is the most wonderful thing that could have happened and the answer to my wishes. Where there was sadness and scars she has helped to bring peace and joy.

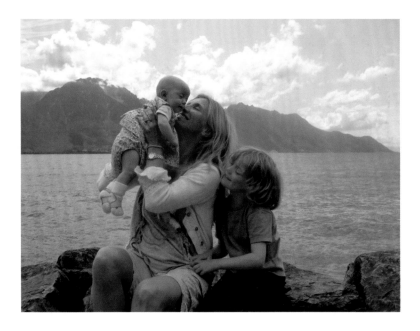

PERSONAL NOTES

References for some insights offered for parts of the information expressed in this book.

Nash, Mike (2nd revised edition 2005) *Aggressive Health*. Milton Keynes. UK: Raw Perfection Ltd

Chopra, Deepack Dr (2nd revised edition 2001) *Perfect Health*. London:Bantam

Servavn-Schreiber, Dr David (2011) *Healing Without Freud or Prozac*. London: Pan Macmillan

Sidhwa, Keki (1994) *The Quintessence of Natural Living for Health and Happiness*. Warwick: British Natural Hygiene Society 1994

TO SEE THE RECIPES AND EXERCISES ONLINE AND CREATE YOUR OWN SHOPPING LIST, SIGN UP AT TIDYTHETEMPLE.COM USING 'TTTFREEBIES'.